Microbiology for GNM

Ashutosh Debata MSc PhD
Director, Dhaneswar Rath Institute of Engineering
and Medical Science
Tangi, Cuttack
Odisha, India

Darshan Panda MSc Microbiology
Research Scholar
Department of Biotechnology
Ravenshaw University, Cuttack
Odisha, India

Sandeep Dhuper MSc Microbiology
Lecturer in Microbiology, LearnEx Academy,
8504 Clearbrook Drive, Fort Worth
Texas, United States

JAYPEE *The Health Sciences Publisher*
New Delhi | London | Philadelphia | Panama

Jaypee Brothers Medical Publishers (P) Ltd

Headquarters

Jaypee Brothers Medical Publishers (P) Ltd
4838/24, Ansari Road, Daryaganj
New Delhi 110 002, India
Phone: +91-11-43574357
Fax: +91-11-43574314
Email: jaypee@jaypeebrothers.com

Overseas Offices

J.P. Medical Ltd
83, Victoria Street, London
SW1H 0HW (UK)
Phone: +44-20 3170 8910
Fax: +44 (0)20 3008 6180
Email: info@jpmedpub.com

Jaypee Medical Inc.
The Bourse
111, South Independence Mall East
Suite 835, Philadelphia, PA 19106, USA
Phone: +1 267-519-9789
Email: joe.rusko@jaypeebrothers.com

Jaypee Brothers Medical Publishers (P) Ltd
Bhotahity, Kathmandu, Nepal
Phone: +977-9741283608
Email: Kathmandu@jaypeebrothers.com

Jaypee-Highlights Medical Publishers Inc
City of Knowledge, Bld. 237, Clayton
Panama City, Panama
Phone: +1 507-301-0496
Fax: +1 507-301-0499
Email: cservice@jphmedical.com

Jaypee Brothers Medical Publishers (P) Ltd
17/1-B, Babar Road, Block-B, Shaymali
Mohammadpur, Dhaka-1207
Bangladesh
Mobile: +08801912003485
Email: jaypeedhaka@gmail.com

Website: www.jaypeebrothers.com
Website: www.jaypeedigital.com

Textbook of Microbiology for GNM Students

First Edition: **2015**

ISBN 978-93-5152-650-6

Printed at: Sterling Graphics Pvt. Ltd.

Dedicated to

In the loving memory of Gold Medalist, Eminient Physician, Doctor's International Awardee and Renowned worker in Freedom struggle, (Late) Dr Baikunthanath Debata of Salipur, Cuttack, seeking his Eternal Blessings.

Preface

Many of the health problems in developing countries like India are different from those of developed countries. Bacterial diseases still play a considerable role in our country. Nurses form the backbone of any medical services or patient care in the health sector. Nursing encompasses autonomous and collaborative care of individuals of all ages, families, groups and communities, sick or well and in all settings. It aims at promotion of health, prevention of illness and the care of ill, disabled and dying people. Knowledge of microbiology is indispensably linked with nursing practice. It is one of the fundamental bases of knowledge that governs how every nurse interacts with patients in many settings. Nurses apply knowledge of microbiology in methods of infection control, keeping instruments clean and free of contamination, how to dress wounds safely in a way that minimizes the possibility of infection, and also in identifying types of infections.

Textbook of Microbiology for GNM Students delves into ever demanding, thoughtful necessity of an absolutely well documented compilation of factual details related to theoretical principles and point wise explanation catering to the needs of GNM students. The entire course content presented in the GNM Microbiology syllabus has been developed meticulously and painstakingly. It has been designed and expanded as per the **Indian Nursing Council (INC) Syllabus.** Each chapter has duly been enumerated in a simple, lucid and crisp language easily comprehensible by its readers. An innovative and widely acceptable style of presentation has been adopted encompassing introduction, labeled diagrams, graphics, descriptions, explanations, possible questions, model answers and suggested reading. It is assumed that this edition will be useful for nursing students and faculties.

Ashutosh Debata
Darshan Panda
Sandeep Dhuper

Acknowledgments

On the eve of the publication of Textbook of Microbiology for GNM Students, we would like to acknowledge the unbound inspiration received from Mr Pramod Chandra Rath, Chairman, DRIEMS Group of Institutions, Tangi, Cuttack; a personality interested in the field of Science and Technology Education that contribute largely in Health Education and Service. We crop up a desire to express our profound gratitude to Hon'ble Justice RK Patra for motivating us incessantly at every step during this venture.

Additionally, we seek to thank Mr Narendra Panda, Mr Abinash Panda, Mr Chetan Dhuper, Dr Abhitosh Debata, Er Arun Panda, Mr Magan Vashisht, Er Sumita Debata for their whole hearted co-operation. We duly accede the enthusiasm of Dr Chinmoy Raj in extending a helping hand for the completion of this edition. We will fail in our duty if we do not express our gratitude to Jaypee Brothers Medical Publishers for the publication of this Textbook.

Contents

GNM Syllabus

Hrs. 30

Course Description

This course is designed to help students gain knowledge and understanding of the characteristics and activities of micro-organisms, how they react under different conditions and how they cause different disorders and diseases. Knowledge of these principles will enable students to understand and adopt practices associated with preventive and promotive health care.

General Objectives

Upon completion of this course, the students will be able to:

1. Describe the classifications and characteristics of microorganisms.
2. List the common disease producing microorganisms and their characteristics.
3. Explain the activities of microorganism in relation to the environment and the human body.
4. Enumerate the basic principle of control and destruction of micro-organisms.
5. Apply the principle of microbiology in nursing practice.

Course Content

Unit I Introduction

Brief historical review of bacteriology and microbiology. Scope and usefulness of knowledge of microbiology in nursing.

Unit II Microorganisms

Classification, structure, size, method and rate of reproduction. Factors influencing growth. Pathogenic and non-pathogenic organisms. Normal flora of the body. Common diseases caused by different types of microorganisms.

Unit III Infection and its Transmission

Sources of infection. Growth of microbes. Portals of entry and exit of microbes. Transmission of infection. Collection of specimens.

Unit IV Immunity

Types of immunity. Hypersensitivity and autoimmunity.

Unit V The Control and Destruction of Microorganisms

Principle and methods of microbial control. Sterilization: dry heat, moist heat, chemicals and radiation. Disinfection physical, natural gases, chemicals used and preparation of lotions. Chemotherapy and antibiotics. Medical and surgical asepsis, cross-infection. Control of spread of infection. Pasteurization Bio-safety and waste management.

Unit VI Introduction to Laboratory Techniques

Microscope: Parts and uses. Handling and care of microscope. Inoculation of culture media. Staining and examination of slides. Preparation and examination of smears.

Plate 1

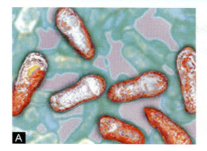
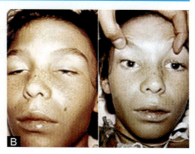
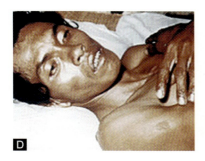
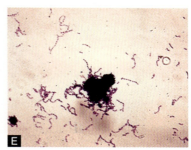
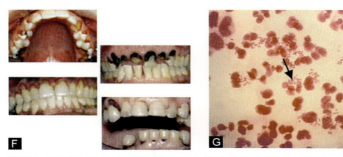

Figures 9.1 (A, B, D to G): Common Bacterial diseases of human beings:
(A) *Clostridium botulinum*, causal organism of botulism, (B) A 14-year-old
patient with botulism, (D) A person with severe dehydration due to cholera,
(E) *Streptococcus mutans*, causal organism of dental caries, (F) Dental caries,
(G) *Neisseria gonorrhoeae*, causal organism of gonorrhoeae

Plate 2

Gonnorhea

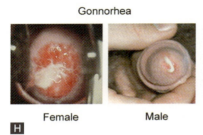

Female   Male

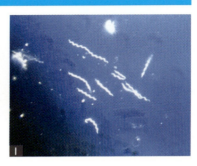

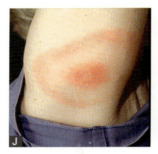

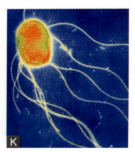

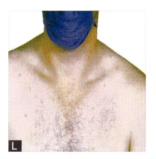

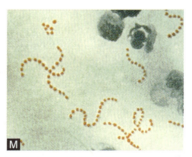

Figures 9.1 (H to M): Common Bacterial diseases of human beings: (H) Gonorrhoeae in male and female, (I) *Borrelia burgdorferi*, causal organism of Lyme disease, (J) Classic bull's-eye appearance is also called erythema migrans, (K) *Salmonella typhi*, causal organism of typhoid, (L) Rose spots on the chest of a patient with typhoid fever due to the bacterium *Salmonella*, (M) *Streptococcus pyogenes*, causal organism of streptococcal pharyngitis

Plate 3

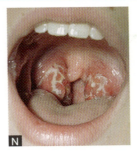

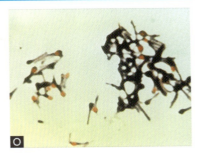

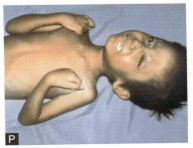

Figures 9.1 (N to P): Common Bacterial diseases of human beings: (N) Streptococcal pharyngitis, (O) *Clostridium tetani*, causal organism of tetanus, (P) A child suffering from tetanus

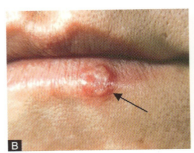

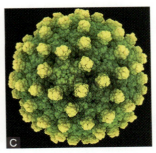

Figures 9.2 (B and C): Common Viral diseases in human beings: (B) Herpes labialis (blister) of the lower lip in a herpes patient, (C) Hepatitis A virus

Plate 4

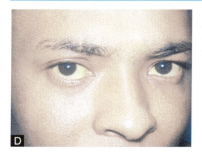

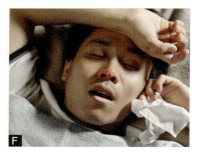

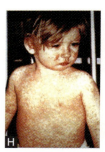

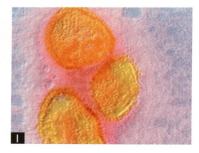

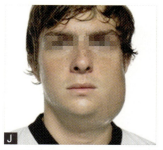

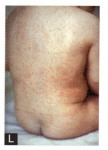

Figures 9.2 (D, F, H to J, L): Common Viral diseases in human beings: (D) A case of jaundice caused by hepatitis A, (F) A patient suffering from Influenza, (H) A patient suffering from measles, (I) Mumps virus, (J) A patient suffering from mumps, (L) A patient suffering from Rubella (German fever)

Plate 5

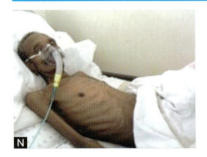
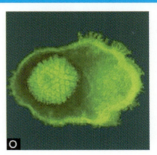

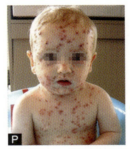

Figures 9.2 (N to P): Common Viral diseases in human beings: (N) A patient suffering from Acquired Immunodeficiency syndrome (AIDS), (O) *Varicella zoaster* virus, (P) A child suffering from small pox.

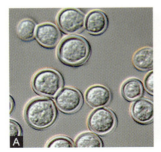
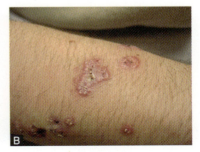

Figures 9.3 (A and B): Mycosis: (A) *Blastomyces dermatitidis*, causal organism of Blastomycosis, (B) Blastomycosis

Plate 6

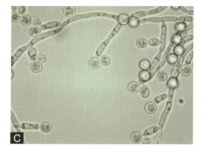

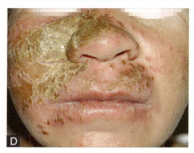

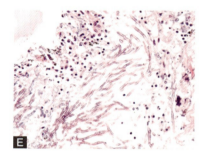

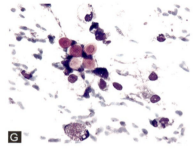

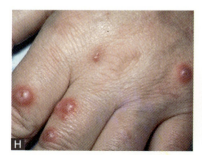

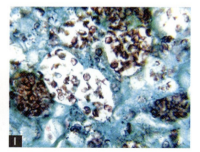

Figures 9.3 (C to E and G to I): Mycosis: (C) *Candida albicans*, Causal organism of Candidiasis, (D) Candidiasis, (E) *Aspergillus* spp., causal organism of Aspergillosis, (G) *Cryptococcus neoformans*, causal organism of Cryptococcosis, (H) Cryptococcosis, (I) *Histoplasma capsulatum*, causal organism of Histoplasmosis

Plate 7

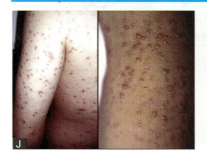
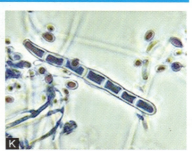

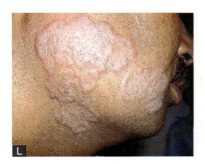
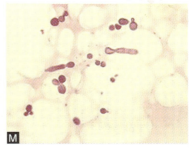

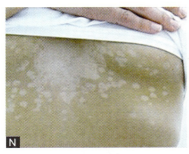
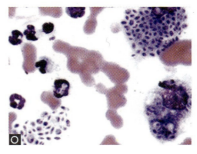

Figures 9.3 (J to O): Mycosis: (J) Colony of *Histoplasma capsulatum* inside the lungs of the patient suffering from Histoplasmosis, (K) *Tricophyton rubrum* (Dermatophyte), causal organisms of Dermatophytosis, (L) Dermatophytosis, (M) *Malassezia furfur*, causal organisms of Tinea versicolor (N) *Tinea versicolor*, (O) *Sporothrix schenckii*, causal organism of Sporotrichosis

Plate 8

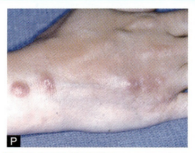

Figure 9.3 (P): Mycosis: (P) Sporotrichosis

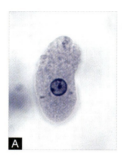

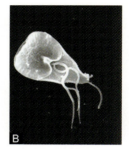

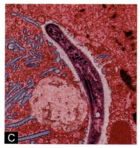

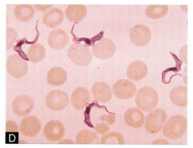

Figures 9.4 (A to D): Common protozoan parasites of human beings: (A) *Entamoeba histolytica*, causal organism of amoebiasis, (B) *Giardia lamblia*, causal organism of giardiasis, (C) *Plasmodium vivax*, causal organism of malaria, (D) *Trypanosoma brucei*, causal organism of African sleeping sickness

Chapter

1

Introduction to Microbiology

■ WHAT ARE MICROORGANISMS?

Microorganisms are microscopic organisms (very small and can only be seen by microscope). These may be unicellular (having a single cell) or multicellular (having more than one cell).

Table 1.1: General characteristics of microorganisms

Characteristics	
Body plan	Single cell or cluster of cells
Organelles	They lack organelles
Size	Dimensions of microscopic organisms fall within the range of micrometers, sometimes nanometers Most microbes extend from the smallest viruses to much bigger protozoans
Habitat	They are ubiquitous (found everywhere)
Classification	They are generally classified as : Archaea, Bacteria, Fungi, Viruses, Protozoa and Algae
Microorganisms to Environment	Microorganisms such as algae produce oxygen. They decompose organic material, provide nutrients for plants, etc.
Microorganisms to Humans	Some microorganisms are good for human health and some are pathogenic (causing severe diseases in human and animals)
Factors affecting Growth of Microorganisms	Nutrients, Oxygen, Water, Temperature, Acidity, Light and Chemicals affect the growth of microorganisms

▮ MICROBIOLOGY: STUDY OF MICROORGANISMS

Microbiology is the Scientific study of microorganisms. Various branches of Microbiology include:

- Bacteriology: the study of bacteria.
- Mycology: the study of fungi.
- Protozoology: the study of protozoa.
- Phycology (or algology): the study of algae.
- Parasitology: the study of parasites.
- Virology: the study of viruses.
- Nematology: the study of the nematodes.

▮ CATEGORIES OF MICROORGANISMS

Depending on their cell type, microorganisms are divided into (Flow chart 1.1);

Eukaryotic Microorganisms

They have complex cellular structure similar to those of human and animals. Their cells have nuclei and mitochondria. They are self-sufficient and capable of leading independent lives.
Examples

- Fungi: Molds and yeasts
- Helminthes: Tape worm, Hooke worms
- Protozoa: *Plasmodium*
- Unicellular Algae: *Chlamydomonas*

Prokaryotic Microorganisms

They are simple, self-sufficient, unicellular organisms having primitive nuclei and mitochondria being capable of leading independent lives.
Examples

- Bacteria: *E.coli, Vibrio cholerae*
- Archaebacteria: *Thermobacillus* SPS
- Cyanobacteria: *Spirulina* SPS

Noncellular Microorganisms

They are without any cell forms and are called as acellular. They are of following types:

- Viruses: They consist of DNA or RNA and proteins. They are not capable of leading independent lives. They grow and multiply by infecting cells of higher organisms (prokaryotic and eukaryotic cells).
- Prions: They are made up of only proteins that cause Bovine Spongiform Encephalopathy (BSE), Kunue, etc.
- Virusoids are madeup of single stranded RNA.
- Viroidis are made-up of circular but single stranded RNA without protein. It causes Viral Hepatitis D

Flowchart 1.1: Categories of microoganisms depending on their cell type

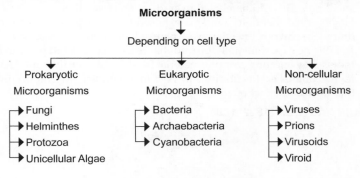

Microorganisms
↓
Depending on cell type

Prokaryotic	Eukaryotic	Non-cellular
Microorganisms	Microorganisms	Microorganisms
➤ Fungi	➤ Bacteria	➤ Viruses
➤ Helminthes	➤ Archaebacteria	➤ Prions
➤ Protozoa	➤ Cyanobacteria	➤ Virusoids
➤ Unicellular Algae		➤ Viroid

◾ HISTORY OF MICROBIOLOGY

It was not very clear that microscopic living organisms exist. In 1600 AD Anton van Leeuwenhoek built his own microscopes and made first detailed descriptions of microscopic living creatures. Leeuwenhoek observed a variety of things like rain water, pond water and scrapings from his own teeth under the lens of his so-called microscope. He saw minute moving objects and called them as "Little animalcules", such as protozoa, yeasts and bacteria. He made accurate sketches and communicated his findings to "Royal Society of London". He had most likely observed single celled eukarytoic microbes. With this observation the Science of Microbiology was started. For this reason Anton van Leeuwenhoek is called as the Father of Microbiology.

◾ CONTRIBUTION OF EMINENT SCIENTISTS TO MICROBIOLOGY

EDWARD JENNER (1749–1823)

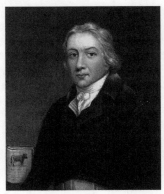

Figure 1.1: Edward Jenner (1749–1823)

- Jenner was an English doctor who discovered vaccination against small pox. This ultimately led to eradication of small pox.
- He observed that dairy workers exposed to occupational (from their dairy job) cowpox infection were naturally immune to small pox.
- In 1796, he experimentally proved that resistance to small pox can be induced by injecting cow pox material from disease pustules into man.
- Jenner published his findings in 1798 in a pamplet "An inquiry into the cause and effect of variole vaccine".

LOUIS PASTEUR (1822–1895)

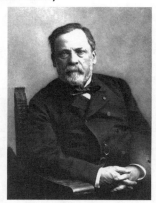

Figure 1.2: Louis Pasteur (1822–1895)

Era	Discoverer	Important Events
Eighteenth Century	Edward Jenner (1729–1799)	Discovery of small pox vaccine
Nineteenth Century	Justus von Liebig (1803–1873)	Conceptualized the physico-chemical theory of fementation
	Ignaz Phillipp Semmelwets (1818–1865)	First and foremost introduced the application of antiseptics.
	Joseph Lister (1827–1912)	Developed aseptic techniques: Isolated bacteria in pure culture.
	Fenny Hesse (1850–1934)	Suggested use of agar as a solidifying material for the preparation of microbiological media.
	Paul Ehrlich (1854–1915)	Developed modern concept of chemotherapy and chemotherapeutic agents.
	Hans Christian Gram (1853–1933)	Invented vital and important procedure for differential staining of microorganisms, i.e. the well-known Gram Stain.

Era	Discoverer	Important Events
Twentieth Century	August von Wassermann (1866–1925)	Developed complement-fixation test for syphillis.
	Martinus Williem Beijerinek (1851–1931)	Employed the principles of enrichment cultures: confirmed finding of the very first virus.
	Felix H.d' Herelle (1873–1949)	Discovered independently the bacteriophages, i.e. viruses that destroy bacteria.

- He was a Professor of Chemistry at the University of Lille, France.
- He is also called as "Father of Modern Microbiology".
- Generation"(Abiogenesis), experimentally by using swan-necked flasks experiment.
- He experimentally showed that souring of wine and beer is due to the growth of undesirable organisms.
- He also showed that the desirable microorganisms produce alcohol by a chemical process called "Fermentation".
- He introduced the technique of "Pasteurization" and proposed the "Germ theory of disease".

Germ Theory of Disease

- This theory was developed in 1860's, by Louis Pasteur.
- It states that tiny living beings are the cause of infectious diseases.
- While doing his research in puerperal fever or child bed fever Louis Pasteur proposed this theory.
- This disease for the first time supports that pathogenic microorganisms such as bacteria and viruses could cause disease.
- The term "germ" here stands for microscopic organisms that cause infectious diseases.
- Apart from the pathogen itself, certain environmental and hereditary factors may cause severity of the disease.

Pasteurization

- This is a special technique of heat sterilization developed by Louis Pasteur.
- Originally it was used to kill undesirable microorganisms that cause souring of wine.
- This technique is now extensively used to kill disease causing germs in milk.
- The process of pasteurization of milk includes heating it to 60–65°C (140–150°F) for 30 mins followed by a rapid cooling.
- This decreases the rapid curdling of milk due to the action of microorganisms.

- He developed **steam sterilization technique,** today popularly called as **autoclaving.**
- **He experimentally** differentiated between aerobic and anaerobic bacteria and coined the term **"anaerobic"** to refer the organisms that do not require oxygen for growth.
- He developed **anthrax vaccine.**
- He also developed a **vaccine against rabies** (Hydrophobia).

ROBERT KOCH (1843–1912)

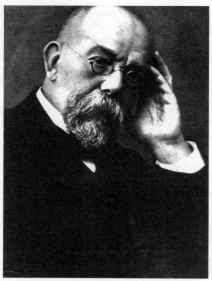

Figure 1.3: Robert Koch (1843–1912)

- He was a German doctor who later became the Professor of hygiene and Director of Institute of Infective Diseases at Berlin.
- He is known as Father of practical bacteriology.
- He is also regarded as "Father of Medical Microbiology and Bacteriology".
- He discovered *Bacillus anthracis,* the causal organism of the disease Anthrax.
- He introduced staining techniques for the study of disease causing microorganisms.
- He discovered *Mycobacterium tuberculosis* which causes Tuberculosis in human beings.
- He also discovered *Vibrio cholerae,* the causative agent of Cholera disease.

- He developed pure culture techniques by introducing solid media.
- He had a great contribution in the development of pure culture techniques.
- He gave Koch's Postulates.

Koch's Postulates

- A specific organism should be found constantly in association with disease.
- The organisms should be isolated and grown in a pure culture in the laboratory.
- The pure culture when incoulated into a healthy susceptible animal should produce symptoms/lesions of the same disease.
- From the inoculated animals, the microorganism should be isolated in pure culture.
- An additional criterion introduced is that specific antiboidies to the causative organisms should be demonstrable in patient's serum.

JOSEPH LISTER (1827–1912)

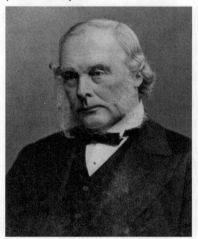

Figure 1.4: Joseph Lister (1827–1912)

- He was a Professor of Surgery at University of Glassglow and Edinburg and later at King's College, London.
- He is also known as "Father of Antiseptic Surgery".
- He was the first person to use an antiseptic solution during the process of surgery.
- He used Carbolic Acid (phenol) on the wound during surgery which successfully prevented sepsis (infection) after operation.
- He also introduced application of carbolic acid during wound dressing.
- Lister's antiseptic surgery later led to the development of aseptic surgery.

ELIE METCHNIKOFF (1845–1916)

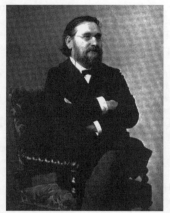

Figure 1.5: Elie Metchnikoff (1845–1916)

- Elie Metchnikoff, a Russian-French Biologist, discovered the phenomenon of phagocytosis.
- He discovered the process of phagocytosis in the transparent larvae of starfish.
- The cells which carry out phagocytosis are called as phagocytes.
- While working at Pasteur Institute in Paris, he found that in human blood leukocytes carry out phagocytosis against invading bacteria.
- Large number of leukocytes gather in the infected area which results in swelling, reddening and pain due to dead phagocytes forming pus.

ALEXANDER FLEMING (1881–1955)

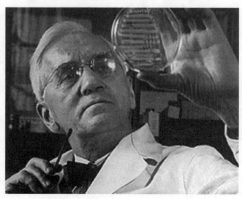

Figure 1.6: Alexander Fleming (1881–1955)

- He was an English Scientist who worked at ST. Marry's hospital in London.
- He discovered lysozyme in 1922 by demonstrating that nasal secretion (fluid from nose) has the power of killing certain bacteria.
- Lysozymes are enzymes present in body fluids such as tears, sweat, and nasal fluid that have the power to kill certain bacteria.
- In 1929, he made an accidental discovery of the antibiotic Penicillin from the fungus Penicillium notatum.
- In 1945 Fleming, Florey and Chain shared the noble prize in physiology and medicine for the discovery of Penicillin.

PAUL EHRLICH (1854–1915)

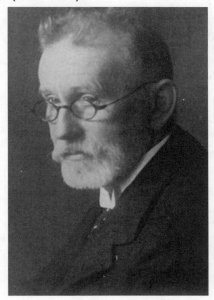

Figure 1.7: Paul Ehrlich (1854–1915)

- He was a German Bacteriologist who invented the technique of Chemotherapy in medicine.
- He is also called as "Father of Chemotherapy".
- The very concept of Chemotherapy is based on the fact that organisms causing diseases could selectively be killed with chemical drugs without harming the host.
- He produced the first synthetic drug – Arsphenamine to control the Syphilis disease.
- He also observed that drug would undergo certain changes in the body after it would produce desired action.

■ POSSIBLE QUESTIONS

1. What is microbiology? Write an essay on the history of microbiology.
2. What are microorganisms? Give an account of their characteristic features.
3. Write Short Notes
   - Louis Pasteur
   - Germ theory of disease
   - Pasteurization
   - Robert Koch
   - Koch's postulates
   - Edward Jenner
   - Joseph Lister
   - Antiseptic Surgery
   - Penicillin
   - Lysozyme
   - Paul Ehrlich

Chapter

2

Scope of Microbiology of Nursing

■ THE PROFESSION OF NURSING

Nursing care focuses on distributing superior quality health care to the patients. This goal requires the nurse to perform following tasks:

- Assessment
- Diagnosis
- Outcome identification
- Planning
- Implementation
- Evaluation

Nurses assess patient's condition by observation, interview and examination of individuals. After collecting the data, nurse analyzes the situation and generates diagnosis. This is the reason why they should have good knowledge in the fundamentals of Microbiology.

■ MEDICAL MICROBIOLOGY

Microorganisms which cause diseases are called as pathogens. Medical microbiology is the branch of Microbiology which carries out study on the pathogens. A Medical microbiologist is an individual who works to;

- study organisms which can cause diseases in people
- look at the life cycle of such organisms
- find out how they cause infections in human
- find out the cause of spread of microorganisms
- find out the effects of microbes on human body
- find out how can microbes be eradicated

■ MICROBIOLOGY IN NURSING

Nursing Microbiology deals with the application of knowledge in Medical Microbiology for nursing care. The principles of personal, hospital and community hygiene are based on the understanding of Microbiology. Nurses play an important role in the field of preventive medicine and healthcare. Microbiology is necessary for nurses in following ways:

- Collect and handle specimen for bacteriological examination
- Understand principles of sterilization and disinfection
- Understand the susceptibility and resistance of microorganisms to drugs
- Learn the process of spread of infection
- Identify pathogenic (disease causing) and non- pathogenic microbes
- Understand the importance of immunity and vaccination
- Interpret reports recovered from laboratories

■ APPLICATION OF MICROBIOLOGY IN NURSING

Followings are important applications of Microbiology in the field of Nursing:

- Nurses use hot water or antiseptic as a measure to sterilize the surgical knives, needles, scissors or any medical equipment to make it free from microbes.
- Microbiology gives knowledge to nurses on how to handle a patient's collected sample infected with communicable diseases.
- If a patient is admitted in hospital and is prescribed an antibiotic which does not found to be effective in him, then it is the duty of the nurse to collect patient's sputum, faecal, urine or blood samples and send it to the laboratory for examination of antibiotic resistance test.
- Nurses carry out blood group tests whenever necessary.
- Nurses carry out different types of diagnostic tests, for example, Mantoux test for Tuberculosis, etc.

■ ROLE OF THE NURSING STAFF IN INFECTION CONTROL

It is the duty of nurses to be familiar with various practices involved in the prevention of the occurrence and spread of infection.

The senior nursing administrator in the hospital is responsible:

- to participate in the hospital infection control committee
- to promote development and improvement of nursing techniques for the maintenance of an aseptic environment in the hospital
- to develop training for the members of nursing staffs in order to educate them in infection control program

The nurse in charge of a ward must have good knowledge in Microbiology for following reasons:

- Maintaining hygiene consistent with hospital policies
- Monitoring aseptic techniques including hand washing
- Shifting infected patient to separate room in order to prevent the spread of disease
- Proper monitoring of the hospital waste

■ POSSIBLE QUESTIONS

1. **What is the scope of microbiology in the field of nursing?**
2. **Write Short Notes**
   - Medical microbiology
   - Nursing microbiology
   - Infection control

Chapter

3

Classification of Microorganisms

■ WHAT IS THE CLASSIFICATION OF MICROORGANISMS?

Biological Classification, or Taxonomy is a method of classifying and categorizing living organisms into groups which share similar characteristic features. There are different types of microorganisms, each differing in its characteristic features. In order to have a systematic study they can be classified under various groups.

■ WHY WE NEED TO CLASSIFY MICROORGANISMS?

More than five million species of microorganisms have already been reported. Thousands more are added to the list every year. It would be difficult to describe and name each one individually. If any microorganism is picked up randomly it would not be possible to describe its basic properties and features so easily. But if their groups are made based on similarities of characteristics then it would be easy to identify them and understand their basic characteristic features.

■ BASIS OF CLASSIFICATION

We classify microorganisms on the following basis:
- Cell type: eukaryotic or prokaryotic
- Cellular or acellular
- Biochemical Properties

■ MAJOR GROUPS OF MICROORGANISMS

Eukaryotic Microorganisms

Basic Features of Eukaryotic cells

- Contain nucleus bounded by nuclear membrane
- Contain complex phospholipids, sphingolipids, histones and sterols

- Have multiple diploid linear (straight) chromosomes and nucleosomes
- Have 80S ribosomes
- Have membrane bound cell organelles such as vacuoles, mitochondria, etc.

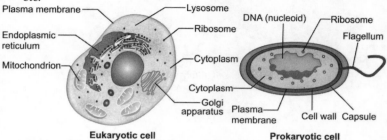

Figure 3.1: Eukaryotic and prokaryotic cells

Followings are types of eukaryotic microorganisms:

Protozoa

- Protozoa are eukaryotic microorganisms.
- Protozoa lack the capability for photosynthesis, although the genus Euglena is renowned for motility as well as carrying out photosynthesis and is therefore considered both as alga and protozoan.
- Although most protozoa reproduce by asexual methods, sexual reproduction has been observed in several species.
- Most protozoa species are aerobic but some anaerobic species have been found in the human intestine and animal lumen.
- Protozoa are located in most moist habitats. Free-living species inhabit freshwater and marine environments and terrestrial species inhabit decaying organic matter. Some species are parasites of plants and animals.
- Protozoa play an important role as **zooplankton,** the free-floating aquatic organisms of the oceans.
- Their cells have no cell walls and therefore can assume an infinite variety of shapes.
- Most protozoa have a single nucleus but some have both macro-nucleus and one or more micronuclei. Contractile vacuoles may be present in protozoa to remove excess water and food vacuoles are often observed.
- Protozoa are **heterotrophic** microorganisms and most species obtain large food particles by **phagocytosis.**
- Many protozoa species move independently by one of three types of locomotor organelles: flagella, cilia and pseudopodia.
- *Example: Entamoeba histolytica* causes amoebiasis in human beings

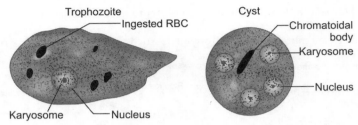

Figure 3.2: *Entamoeba histolytica*, the causal agent of amoebiasis in human beings

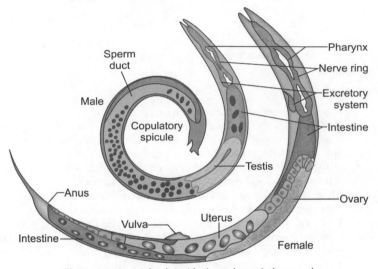

Figure 3.3: *Ascaris lumbrieoides* (roundworm), the causal agent of Ascariasis in humans

Helminths

- Helminths are parasitic, multicellular eukaryotic animals.
- The majority of these animals belong to phyla Platyhelminthes and Nematoda.
- Many parasitic helminths do not have a digestive system and instead absorb nutrients from the food that is consumed by their host organisms, the host's body fluids and tissues.
- Parasitic helminths have very simple nervous system because they have to respond to very few changes in their host's environment.
- They lack or have reduced means of locomotion because they are transferred from one host to another.
- Parasitic helminths have complex reproductive system that produces fertilized eggs (zygotes) which infect the host organism.

- *Examples:*
  - *Taenia solium* (Pork tapeworm) causes Taeniasis
  - *Ascaris lumbrieoides* (roundworm) causes Ascariasis

Fungi

- Fungi are **eukaryotic** and have membrane-bound cellular organelles and nuclei.
- They have no plastids of any kind (and no chlorophyll). The hyphae of fungi are of two general kinds: Some are **septate** and are divided by **septa** (walls) that separate cylindrical hyphae into cells; in **nonseptate** fungi, the hypha is one long tube.
- Mitosis occurs in nonseptate hyphae, but there is no accompanying **cytokinesis** (division of the cytoplasm) so the hyphae are **multinucleate** (with many nuclei).

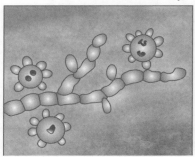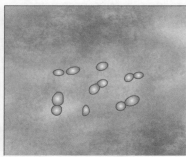

Figure 3.4: *Histoplasma capsulatum*, the causal agent of histoplasmosis in human beings

- An organism or part of an organism with many nuclei not separated by walls or membranes—is termed as **coenocytic** and the organism is a coenocyte.
- Fungi are **heterotrophic** but unlike animals and many other heterotrophs can ingest their nutrients as bits or bites of food, the fungi secrete digestive enzymes into their surroundings and in effect digesting their food outside of their bodies.
- They can absorb smaller particles and incorporate nutrients into their own cells. Some are **parasites** obtaining nutrients from living organisms but more are **saprobes (saprotrophs)** that digest and recycle materials from dead organisms.
- *Example: Histoplasma capsulatum* causes histoplasmosis in human beings

Algae

- **Algae** are eukaryotic organisms that have no roots, stems, or leaves but do have chlorophyll and other pigments for carrying out photosynthesis.

- Algae may be unicellular or multicellular.
- **Unicellular algae** occur most frequently in water especially in plankton.
- **Phytoplankton** is the population of free floating microorganisms composed primarily of unicellular algae.
- Algae establish symbiosis with fungi to form lichen.
- Reproduction in algae occurs in both asexual and sexual forms. Asexual reproduction occurs through fragmentation of colonial and filamentous algae or by spore formation (as in fungi). Spore formation takes place by mitosis. Binary fission also occurs (as in bacteria).
- *Example: Prototheca cutis* causes skin infection in human beings

Prokaryotic Microorganisms

Basic Features of Prokaryotic cells

- Lack nuclei.
- Have single circular chromosome. Some also contain plasmids.
- Have 70s ribosomes.
- Lack membrane bound cell organelles such as vacuoles, mitochondrias, etc.
- Bacteria
    - Bacteria are prokaryotic organisms.
    - They are microscopic, unicellular, may occur singly or in aggregations to form colonies.
    - They possess rigid cell walls. **Cell wall** is made up of **peptidoglycan (Mureins) and Lipopolysaccharides.**
    - **Ribosomes** are scattered in cytoplasmic matrix and are of **70S type.**
    - Most of the bacteria are heterotrophic. Some bacteria are autotrophic, possess **bacteriochlorophyll** which is not in plastids and instead it is found to be scattered.
    - Motile bacteria possess one or more **flagella.**
    - The common method of multiplication is **binary fission.**
    - True sexual reproduction is lacking but **genetic recombination** occurs by conjugation, transformation and transduction.
    - *Examples:*
        - *Vibrio cholerae* causes Cholera
        - *Salmonella typhi* causes Typhoid
        - *Mycobacterium tuberculosis* causes Tuberculosis

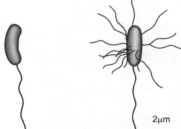

Figure 3.5: *Vibrio cholerae*, the causal agent of Cholera in human beings

Some special categories of Bacteria are :

Chlamydia

- – Chlamydia are Gram-negative bacteria.
- – They are obligate intracellular parasites. They can survive only by establishing "residence" inside the infected cells.
- – They need their host's ATP as energy source for their own cellular activity.
- – They are coccoid in shape and non-motile.
- – They can be transmitted from person to person contact or by airborne respiration.
- – *Examples:*
  - ⁻ *Chlamydia trachomatis* causes trachoma
  - ⁻ *C. pneumoniae causes* mild form of pneumonia in adolescence
  - ⁻ *C. psittaci* causes psittacosis

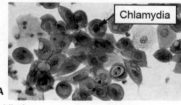

A

How trachoma blinds

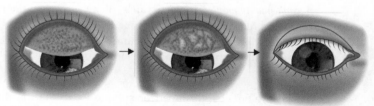

B Infections inflame and thicken the upper eyelid | Scarred eyelids turn inward | The lashes scratch the cornea, leading to blindness

Figures 3.6 A and B: *Chlamydia trachomatis,* the causal agent of trachoma in human beings

Mycoplasma

- The Mycoplasma are tiny free-living organisms capable of self-replication.
- They are smaller than some of larger viruses.
- They lack cell walls.
- Are only prokaryotes that contain sterols.
- They are facultatively anaerobic bacteria.
- Take on many shapes (pleomorphic).
- Mycoplasmas can also resemble fungi because some Mycoplasmas produce filaments that are commonly seen in fungi. It is these filaments that led scientists to name it Mycoplasma. Myco means "fungus."
- Mycoplasma are unable to move by themselves because they do not have flagella but some are able to glide on a wet surface.

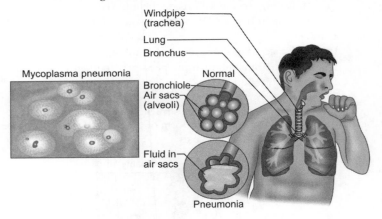

Figure 3.7: *Mycoplasma pneumonia*, the causal agent of a typical pneumonia in human beings

Examples:

- *Mycoplasma pneumonia* is the cause of atypical pneumonia commonly referred to as walking pneumonia
- *Ureaplasma urealyticum* is a bacterium that is found in urine and one that can cause urinary tract infection.

Rickettsia

- Rickettsias are small rod-shaped or spherical bacteria that live in the cells of ticks, lice, fleas, mites (arthropods) and can be transmitted to humans when bitten by arthropods.

- They are small, Gram-negative, non-motile, rod to coccoid-shaped bacteria.
- Rickettsias reproduce by binary fission.
- It is similar to Chlamydia in that they both are of the size of large viruses.
- Like Chlamydia they are obligate intracellular parasites who can't produce ATP and depend for the same on attacked host cell.

Examples:
  - *Rickettsia prowazekii* is transmitted by lice and causes endemic typhus.
  - *R. rickettsii* is transmitted by ticks and causes Rocky Mountain spotted fever.

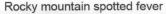

Rocky mountain spotted fever

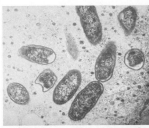

Electron microscopy of
rickettsia rickettsii

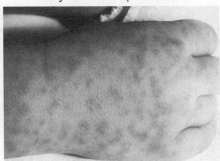

Figure 3.8 *R. Rickettsii*, the causal agent of Rocky Mountain spotted fever in human beings

Siprochaetes

- Spirochaetes are tiny Gram-negative organisms that look like corkscrews.
- They move in a unique spinning motion via 6 thin endoflagella called axial filaments.
- These organisms replicate by transverse fission.
- They cannot be cultured in ordinary media.
- They are too small to be seen using light microscope. Special procedures are required to view these organisms, including darkfield microscopy, immunofluorescence and silver stains.
- *Examples:*
  - *Treponema pallidum* causes Syphilis
  - *Borrelia burgdorferi* causes Lyme disease

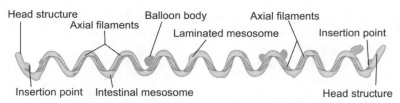

Figure 3.9: *Treponema pallidum*, the causal agent of syphilis

Archaebacteria

- Cell wall is not made up of peptidoglycan.
- Cell membrane contains long-chain branched alcohols (phytanols) bound to glycerol by ethereal linkages.
- They are extremophiles as they can grow in extreme habitats such as at high temperature, under high pressure.
- The major categories of archaebacteria comprise essentially of:
  - *Methanogenic bacteria:* example, *Methanococcus*
  - *Extreme halophiles:* example, *Halobacterium*
  - *Thermophiles:* example, *Thermoplasma*
  - *Acidophiles:* example, *Sulfolobus*

Acellular Microorganisms

Basic Features of Acellular Microbes

- these are neither prokaryotic nor eukaryotic
- do not contain cell wall, cell membrane of any cell organelles
- do not behave as living organisms outside the host cells
- they are made-up of nucleic acid and protein (e.g. virus), only nucleic acid (e.g. viroids) or only protein (e.g. prions)

Viruses

- are acellular and are not visible with light microscope.
- are obligate intracellular parasites.
- contain no organelles or biosynthetic machinery except for few enzymes.
- contain either RNA or DNA as genetic material.
- are called as bacteriophages (or phages) if they have bacterial host.
- Examples:
  - Poxviridae causes pox (pus-filled lesions) diseases such as smallpox
  - Poliovirus causes Poliomyelitis

- Human Immunodeficiency Virus (HIV) causes Acquired Immuno Deficiency Syndrome (AIDS)

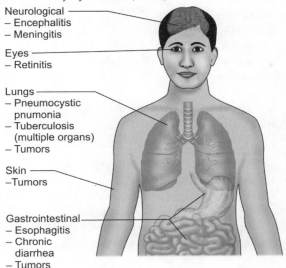

Neurological
– Encephalitis
– Meningitis

Eyes
– Retinitis

Lungs
– Pneumocystic pnumonia
– Tuberculosis (multiple organs)
– Tumors

Skin
–Tumors

Gastrointestinal
– Esophagitis
– Chronic diarrhea
– Tumors

Figure 3.10: Symptoms of AIDS

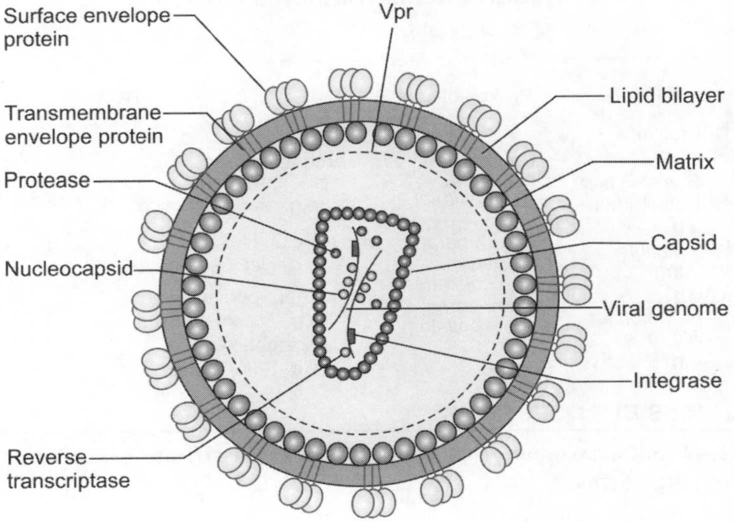

Surface envelope protein

Vpr

Transmembrane envelope protein

Protease

Nucleocapsid

Reverse transcriptase

Lipid bilayer

Matrix

Capsid

Viral genome

Integrase

Figure 3.11: HIV, causal agent of AIDS

Prions

- are infectious particles associated with diseases of the central nervous system.
- are made of proteins only.
- diseases caused by prions are:
  - Scrapie disease in sheep and goats
  - Bovine spongiform encephalopathy ('mad cow disease') in cows
  - Kuru disease in humans (cannibals)
  - Creutzfeldt-Jakob disease in humans

Viroids

- are not cells and not visible with light microscope.
- are obligate intracellular parasites.
- are single-stranded, covalently closed, circular RNA molecules that exist as base-paired, rod like structures.
- cause plant diseases but have not been proven to cause human disease, although the RNA of Hepatitis D virus (HDV) is viroid-like.

Flowchart 3.1: Classification of microorganisms

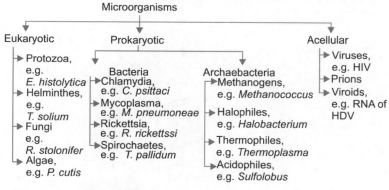

■ POSSIBLE QUESTIONS

1. **What is taxonomy? Give an account of classification of micro-organisms.**

2. **Write Short Notes:**
   - Parasites
   - Tape worm
   - Protozoa
   - Viruses
   - Prions
   - Extremophiles
   - Lichens
   - Viroids
   - Rocky mountain spotted fever
   - Mycoplasma
   - Spirochaete
   - Rickettsia
   - Saprophytes

Chapter

4

Structure of Microorganisms

■ WHAT ARE BACTERIA?

Bacteria (sing: bacterium) are the most well known microorganisms. These are microscopic, prokaryotic, unicellular organisms found everywhere.

■ DISTRIBUTION OF BACTERIA

Bacteria are found in every habitat starting from soil to volcanic zone. They are present in invisible form in the objects we touch, the food we eat, air we breathe, water we drink and from soil to volcanoes. They are found in plants, animals including human beings. The human mouth itself contains 500 species of bacteria. It has been estimated that a single teaspoon of fertile top soil contains more than a billion bacteria.

■ SIZE

Bacterial cells are extremely small. They vary in length and width. The size of bacteria is scientifically measured in the unit 'micron'. Bacteria range in size from 0.2 – 2 microns in width and 1–10 microns in length. It is important to know that bacteria have high surface: volume ratio.

Biggest Bacteria: *Thiomargrita namibiensis*: 100–300 µm

Smallest Bacteria: *Mycoplasma*: 0.2–0.3 µm

■ SHAPE

There are three basic shapes of bacteria viz. Coccus, Bacillus and Spiral:

Table 4.1: Types of bacteria on the basis of their shape

Coccus (Pleural-Cocci): They may be oval or flattened on one side. They can be of following types:			
Diplococci	Cocci that remain in pair	*Diplococcus pneumonae*	Plane of division Diplococci $\vdash$ 2µm $\dashv$
Streptococci	Cocci that remain in chain	*Streptococcus pneumoniae*	Plane of division Streptococci $\vdash$ 2µm $\dashv$
Tetrad	Cocci that remain in a group of 4	*Tessaracoccus bendigoensis*	Tetrad $\vdash$ 1µm $\dashv$
Sarcinae	Cocci that remain in group of 8 to form a cube like structure	*Sarcina ventriculi*	Sarcinae $\vdash$ 2µm $\dashv$
Staphylococci	Cocci that remain in clusters	*Staphylococcus aureus*	Staphylococci $\vdash$ 2µm $\dashv$
Bacillus (Pleural- Bacilli)			
These are of following types:			
Diplobacilli	Bacilli appearing in pair	*Diplobacillus* species	Single bacillus Diplobacilli $\vdash$ 2µm $\dashv$

Cont...

Cont...

Streptoba-cilli	Bacilli that appear in chain	*Streptobacillus moniliformis*	2µm
Cocco bacilli	Bacilli which are short fat and look like cocci	*Acetobacter*	Coccobacillus 1µm

Spiral Bacteria
These are spiral in shape and are of following types:

Vibrio	Look like curved rods	*Vibrio*	Vibrio 2µm
Spirillum	Have helical shape and rigid body	*Borrelia*	Spirillum 2µm
Spirochaete	Have helical shape and flexible body	*Leptospira*	Spirochete 5µm

Other shapes

Stellar bacteria	Star shaped bacteria	*Simonsiella*	
Rectangular bacteria	They are rectangular in shape	*Haloarcula* species	LM 0.5 µm

■ ULTRASTRUCTURE OF BACTERIAL CELL

Bacteria are prokaryotic by their cellular constitution. The parts of bacterial cells are:

(a) Capsule and Slime layer
(b) Cell wall
(c) Cell membrane
(d) Cytoplasm
(e) Chromosome
(f) Plasmids
(g) Ribosomes
(h) Locomotory organs
(i) Inclusion bodies
(j) Pilli and Fimbriae
(k) Endospore

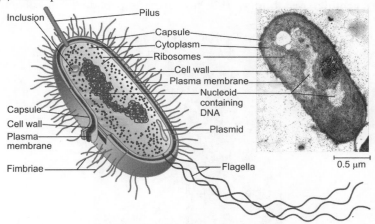

Figure 4.1: Ultrastructure of bacterial cell

(a) Capsule and Slime Layer

Location: A loose coating called Slime layer is usually deposited around the bacterial cell wall. In some bacteria Slime layers become thick and forms capsule.

Structure and Composition: It is made-up of polysaccharides, lipids and proteins.

Function: It helps bacteria to attach on a particular surface. In some pathogenic bacteria (diseases causing bacteria), capsule protects bacterial cell from immune system of the host.

(b) Cell Wall

Location: It is present next to capsule. In some bacterial cells where capsule is absent, cell wall acts as the outermost covering.

Thickness: Gram-Positive Bacteria – 20–80 nm

Gram-Negative Bacteria – 2–3 nm

Structure and Composition: It is made-up of peptidoglycan which differs in two groups of bacteria, namely Gram-negative and Gram-positive. The properties of peptidoglycan are:

- **Polysaccharide backbone:** Consists of two alternating repeating sugars: NAG (N-Acetyl Glucosamine) and NAMA (N-Acetyl Muramic Acid).
- **Tetra peptide:** It is hung from polysaccharide backbone having Amino acids such as L-Alanine, D-Glutamic acid, D-Lysine and D-Alanine. (Note: D type Amino acids are very rare in living organisms).
- **Peptide cross bridge:** This link connects peptidoglycan subunits together.

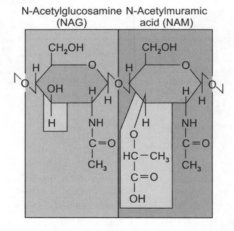

Figure 4.2: Peptidoglycan subunit comprising of N-Acetylglucosamine (NAG) and N-Acetylmuramic Acid (NAM)

Function: It protects the cell from Osmotic shock and physical damage. It also provides rigidity and shape to bacterial cells.

Table 4.2: Difference between Gram-positive and Gram-negative bacteria

Characteristic	Gram-Positive	Gram-Negative
Gram Reaction	Retain crystal violet dye and stain blue or purple	Can be decolorized to accept counterstain (safranin) and stain pink or red
Peptidoglycan Layer	Thick (multilayered)	Thin (single-layered)
Teichoic Acids	Present in many	Absent
Periplasmic Space	Absent	Present
Outer Membrane	Absent	Present
Lipopolysaccharide (LPS) Content	Visually none	High
Lipid and Lipoprotein Content	Low (acid-fast bacteria have lipids linked to peptidoglycan)	High (because of presence of outer membrane)
Flagellar Structure	2 rings in basal body	4 rings in basal body
Toxins Produced	Exotoxins	Endotoxins and Exotoxins
Resistance to Physical Disruption	High	Low
Cell Wall Disruption by Lysozyme	High	Low (acid-fast bacteria have lipids linked to Peptidoglycan)
Susceptibility to Penicillin and Sulfonamide	High	Low
Susceptibility to Streptomycin, Chloramphenicol, and Tetracycline	High	High
Inhibition by Basic Dyes	High	Low
Susceptibility to Anionic Detergents	High	Low
Resistance to Sodium salt	High	Low
Resistance to Drying	High	Low

(c) Cell Membrane

It is also called as Cytoplasmic membrane or Plasma membrane.

Location: It is present next to the cell wall and encloses cytoplasm.

Structure and Composition: The cell membrane is made up of Phospholipid bilayer (two layers of phospholipid molecules) having thickness of 6-8 nm. A phospholipid molecule consists of one hydrophilic (water loving) phosphate group and two hydrophobic (water hating) Fatty Acid chains. Hydrophillic heads are exposed to external environment or cytoplasm. The Fatty Acid chains direct inwards, facing each other due to hydrophobic effects (staying away from water).

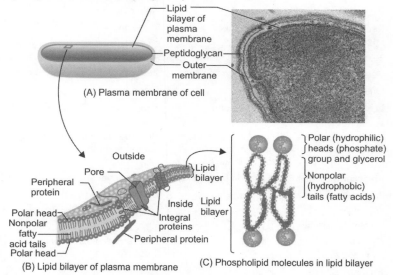

(A) Plasma membrane of cell

(B) Lipid bilayer of plasma membrane

(C) Phospholipid molecules in lipid bilayer

Figures 4.3 (A to C): (A) Plasma membrane of cell, (B) Lipid bilayer of plasma membrane (C) Phospholipid molecules in lipid bilayer

Apart from phospholipids three types of proteins are present in the cell membrane.

- Integral proteins firmly inserted in the membrane. These are mainly involved in transportation and are of three types- uniport, symport and antiport.

- Outer Surface proteins usually present in Gram-negative bacteria. These interact with periplasmic proteins for the transport of large molecules in the cell.

- Inner Surface proteins interact with other proteins in energy producing reactions and other important cellular functions.

- Mesosome: These are infoldings formed by the plasma membrane. These are commonly found in Gram-positive bacteria and play important roles in cell division and replication.

Function: Regulates the specific transport of substances between the cells and outer environment.

(d) Cytoplasm

Location: It is present next to the cell membrane and fills entire inner space of the cell.

Composition: It is a semifluid substance enclosed by the cell membrane. It appears granular due to the presence of large number of ribosomes. Different structures such as chromosomes, plasmids as well as cytoplasmic organelles are found in the cytoplasm.

Note: Membrane bound cell organelles like mitochondria, chloroplasts, lysosomes, golgi complex, vacuoles and endoplasmic reticulum are absent in bacterial cell.

Function: It is the site for various biochemical reactions and contains genetic material of the cell.

(e) Chromosome

The space where the chromosome resides is called as **Nucleoid**.

Location: Since the bacterial cell is prokaryotic, a membrane bound nucleus is absent. Bacterial chromosome is found to float freely in the cytoplasm.

Number: One chromosome in each cell.

Size: In *E.coli* the size of chromosome is 4640 kilo base pairs (kbp).

Structure and Composition: It is made up of circular DNA attached at a point to the plasma membrane. The DNA in bacterial cell is not associated with histone protein. The DNA molecule is composed of nitrogen bases (Adenine, Guanine, Cytosine, Thymine), deoxyribose sugar and phosphate molecules.

Function: It is the storehouse of genetic information.

(f) Plasmid

Apart from chromosomes, certain bacterial cells contain additional DNA molecule called as **plasmid**.

Location: Bacterial plasmid is found to float freely in the cytoplasm.

Number: Present from one to several in number.

Size: Plasmids are much smaller than chromosomes.

Structure and Composition: It is a circular DNA molecule without histones. The plasmid DNA replicates independently.

Function: It contains some special genes such as Fertility factor (F-Factor), Resistance factor (R-Factor), Nitrogen fixing genes (Nif genes). Due to the presence of plasmid bacterial cells get special characteristics.

Note: Some plasmids may temporarily become associated with Nucleoid DNA and are called as Episomes.

(g) Ribosomes

Location: These are evenly distributed in the cytoplasm.

Structure and Composition: Bacteria contain 70S Ribosome and is made up of ribosomal RNA (rRNA) and proteins. 70S Ribosome has two subunits-

- 30S subunit: It has 21 proteins and 16S rRNA.
- 50S subunit: It has 34 proteins, 23S rRNA and 5S rRNA.

Note: "S" stands for Svedburg unit, which represents how rapidly particles or molecules sediment in an ultra centrifuge.

Function: These are involved in bacterial protein synthesis

(h) Locomotory Organs (Flagella and Cilia)

There are two types of locomatory organs in bacteria—the bigger one are called as flagella and the smaller one are called as cilia. Locomatory organs help in the movement or locomotion of bacterial cells. Depending on the presence or absence of locomotory organs bacteria are of two types-

- **Motile:** bacteria that can move, e.g. *Vibrio cholerae*
- **Non-Motile:** Bacteria that cannot move, e.g. *Staphylococcus aureus*

Location: It is present in outer surface of the cell.

Monotrichous	A single flagellum present at one pole of the bacterial cell	*Vibrio*	
Amphitrichous	Each pole of bacteria having one single flagellum		
Cephalotrichous	Each pole having a bunch of flagellae		
Lophotrichous	Bunch of flagellae present at one pole in bacterium	*Thio-spirillum*	
Peritrichous	Flagella evenly distributed throughout the surface of the bacterial cell	*Salmonella typhii*	
Atrichous	Flagella is totally absent in such bacteria	*Staphylococcus*	

Structure and Composition

Flagella are made up of protein called as flagellin. The structure of flagella is divided into three parts:

- Filament: consists of flagellin protein.
- Hook: Single type of protein that connects filament to basal body.
- Basal body: Supports the filament at the base.

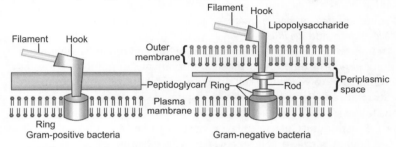

Figure 4.4: Flagella structure in Gram-positive and Gram-negative bacteria

Function: The primary function of flagella is to make bacteria move. There are three types of movement seen:

Chemotaxis: Movement of bacteria towards or away from chemical stimuli.

Magnetotaxis: Movement along the earth's magnetic field.

Phototaxis: Movement of bacteria towards light of different intensities.

(i) Inclusion Bodies

Location: Distributed in the cytoplasm.

These are non-living components present in the cell which do not possess metabolic activity. The most common inclusion bodies are glycogen, lipid droplets, crystals, pigments, volutin granules and metachromatic granules.

(j) Pilli and Fimbrae

Location: Distributed outside the cell surface.

Structure and Composition

Pilli	Fimbrae
Pilli are short, thin, straight, hair like projections composed of protein pilin, carbohydrate and phosphates.	Similar to Pilli but more in number.

Function:

Pilli	Fimbrae
Surface adhesion	Surface adhesion
Sex Pilli participate in genetic material exchange between mating bacterial cells	Formation of biofilm

(k) Endospore

Some species of bacteria are capable of producing endospores, e.g. *Clostridium* and *Bacillus*.

Definition: It is a heat resistant structure that can retain its viability over long period of time under harsh environmental conditions. It can later germinate to a vegetative cell upon the arrival of favorable conditions.

Structure and Composition: An endospore has several coatings which are as follows:

- **Exosporium:** Outermost layer consisting of proteins
- **Spore Coat:** Several layers of spore specific proteins
- **Cortex:** Loosely crossing peptidoglycan
- **Core:** Consists of core wall, cell membrane, cytoplasm, nucleoid, ribosomes and other cellular components.

Function: It helps bacteria to survive during unfavorable environmental conditions.

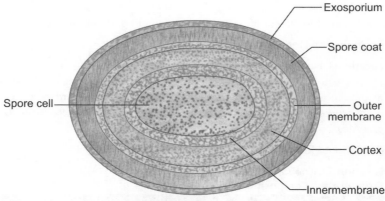

Figure 4.5: Bacterial endospore

■ POSSIBLE QUESTIONS:

1. **Define bacteria. Give a detail account of the ultra structure of a bacterial cell.**

2. **Write Short Notes:**
   - Shape of bacteria
   - Endospore
   - Peptidoglycan
   - Inclusion bodies
   - Nucleoid
   - Plasmid
   - Motility
   - Membrane protein
3. **Differentiate between the following:**
   - Gram-negative and Gram-positive bacteria
   - Capsule and slime layer
   - Pilli and fimbrae
   - Flagella and cilia
   - Plasmid and chromosome

Chapter

5

Microbial Reproduction

■ WHAT IS REPRODUCTION ?

All living things have the ability to reproduce. Reproduction is the process of generating offsprings. Microorganisms also reproduce by various methods in order to increase population. There are two main types of reproduction: Sexual reproduction and asexual reproduction. Some living Organisms reproduce by only one method and others can reproduce using either method. Microorganisms can reproduce sexually and asexually. Microbes have an enormous population because they can reproduce quickly and in so many different ways.

■ TYPES OF REPRODUCTION IN MICROORGANISMS

Asexual Reproduction

It is a type of reproduction where cells from only one parent are used. Only genetically identical organisms are produced by this type of reproduction.

In this Type of Reproduction

- Donor (one which gives DNA) and recipient (one which receives DNA) cells are absent
- Exchange of genetic material (DNA) does not take place
- The offsprings are exact copies of Mother cell

Types of Asexual Reproduction

(a) Budding

In this type of reproduction a small projection, called bud, develops at one end of the cell and one copy of the genetic material gets into the bud. Then the bud enlarges to form a new cell and gets separated from the parent cell.

It Takes Place in following Steps

- Parent cell gives rise to a lateral outgrowth called as bud.
- The chromossome of parent cell is duplicated and passes into the daughter cell.
- The bud grows in size while being attached to the parent body.
- It then gets separated from the parent by the formation of a wall.
- Thereafter the bud falls off and germinates into new individual.
- Thus budding results in formation of daughter cells of unequal size that later grow to adult bodies.

Example: Budding is found in Planctomyces and Yeasts.

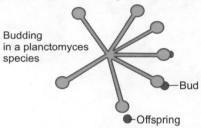

Budding in a planctomyces species

Bud

Offspring

Figure 5.1: Binary fission

(b) Binary Fission

Binary fission generally takes place in bacteria. It is a simple process where the cell increases in size and a double wall develops across the midline of enlarged cell. The enlarged cell then gets separated to form two new cells. Each cell is able to function independently. The process of this type of multiplication in microorganisms is quite rapid. *E. coli* bacterium can double in every 20 minutes at favourable environmental conditions.

It Occurs Through following Steps

- Parental cell enlarges and duplicates its chromosome
- Septum formation (midline wall formation) divides the cell into two separate chambers
- The duplicated chromosome moves to newly formed chamber
- Complete division results in two identical cells
- Each new cell has an identical copy of DNA
- Example, mostly seen in Bacteria

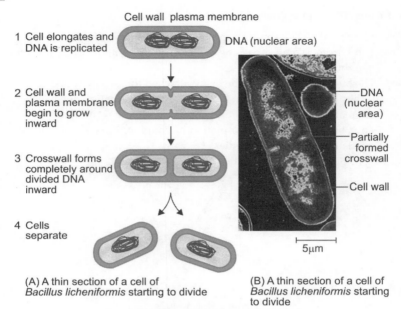

(A) A thin section of a cell of *Bacillus licheniformis* starting to divide

(B) A thin section of a cell of *Bacillus licheniformis* starting to divide

Figures 5.2 (A and B): Endospore formation

(c) Spore Formation or Sporulation

The process of endospore formation in bacteria is called sporulation. During unfavourable condition bacteria produce endospores through following steps:

- **Step 1:** DNA is replicated.
- **Step 2:** DNA aligns along the cell's long axis.
- **Step3:** Cytoplasmic membrane invaginates to form forespore.
- **Step 4:** Cytoplasmic membrane grows and engulfs forespore within a second membrane. The DNA of vegetative cells disintegrates.
- **Step 5:** A cortex of Calcium and Dipicolinic acid is deposited between the membranes.
- **Step 6:** Spore coat forms around endospore.
- **Step 7:** Endospore matures.
- **Step 8:** Endopore releases from the Original cell.

Example: It is seen in Bacteria such as *Bacillus* and *Clostridium*.

(d) Conidia Formation

It takes place in some bacterial and fungal cells. Mostly during unfavourable conditions, bacterial protoplasm divides into small compartments and then gets fragmentized forming minute bodies called as conidia. When the favourable condition arrives, each conidium develops itself into a new bacterium. Each conidium gets a copy of the genetic material.

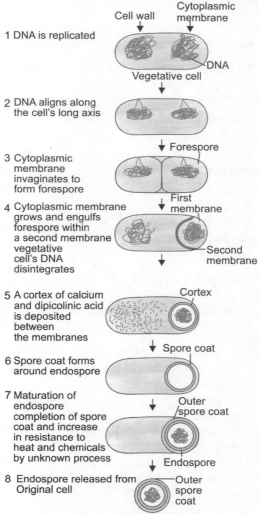

1 DNA is replicated

2 DNA aligns along the cell's long axis

3 Cytoplasmic membrane invaginates to form forespore

4 Cytoplasmic membrane grows and engulfs forespore within a second membrane vegetative cell's DNA disintegrates

5 A cortex of calcium and dipicolinic acid is deposited between the membranes

6 Spore coat forms around endospore

7 Maturation of endospore completion of spore coat and increase in resistance to heat and chemicals by unknown process

8 Endospore released from Original cell

Cell wall

Cytoplasmic membrane

DNA

Vegetative cell

Forespore

First membrane

Second membrane

Cortex

Spore coat

Outer spore coat

Endospore

Outer spore coat

Figure 5.3: Endospore formation by bacteria

(e) Zoospores

This is a common method of asexual reproduction in *Rhizobium* which produces flagellated zoospores.

(f) Cyst

In some bacteria, thick walled spores, similar to endospores are formed. These are called as cysts.

Example: Azotobacter

(g) Fragmentation

It is mostly seen in fungi. In this process the mycelium (fungal filament) breaks into two or more similar fragments either accidentally or due to some external force and each fragment grows into a new fungal filament.

Sexual Reproduction

During Sexual reproduction, two cells, one from each parent, fuse to form a new organism.

In this type of Reproduction

- Donor (one which gives DNA) and recipient (one which receives DNA) cells are present
- Exchange of genetic material (DNA) takes place

Types of Sexual Reproduction

(a) Conjugation

Definition: Conjugation is the process of direct transfer of DNA from one bacterial cell to another bacterial cell. The transferred DNA is a plasmid i.e. a circle of DNA that is distinct from the main bacterial chromosome.

Basic Concept: To understand the steps of conjugation in bacteria one must know different related terms like:

- **F-plasmid:** It is a special plasmid called as Fertility. Plasmid present in some bacterial cell.
- **Donor:** The bacteria which contain the F–plasmid are called as F^+ cells or donor cells.
- **Recipient:** The bacteria which lack the F–plasmid are called as F^- cells or recipient cells.
- **Sex pilus:** This is a specialized thread like structure present on the outer most surface of donor cells (F^+ cells).

Steps of Conjugation

- **Step 1:** Donor cell is attached to a recipient cell with its pilus. The pilus draws the cell together.
- **Step 2:** The cells contact with one another.

- **Step 3:** One strand of F-plasmid DNA is transferred to the recipient
- **Step 4:** The recipient which was F⁻ before, becomes F⁺ after getting the F–plasmid.

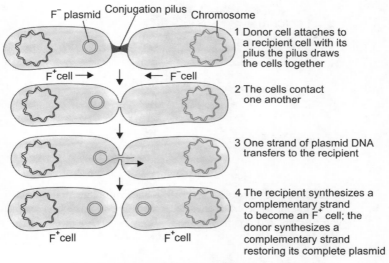

Figure 5.4: Conjugation between F⁺ and F⁻ beacterial cell

(b) Transduction

Definition: Transduction is the process of DNA transfer from one bacterium (donor) to another (recipient) mediated by a virus called as bacteriophage. The recipient cell of a transduction process is called as transductant.

Basic Concept: To understand the steps of conjugation in bacteria one needs to know following terms:

- **Bacteriophage:** It is a virus that attacks bacteria, multiplies inside it and finally kills it. Bacteriophage, like all other viruses, are made-up of nucleic acid and protein. The structure of a bacteriophage is as below:
  - **Nucleic Acid:** The Nucleic acid present in bacteriophage is Deoxyribo Nucleic Acid (DNA). It carries all information (genetic information) which are necessary to carry out the lytic cycle.
  - **Protein Part:** Apart from DNA, all other parts of bacteriophage such as capsid head, collar, sheath, baseplate, spikes and tail fibres are made-up of proteins.

  Example of a bacteriophage is a T4 phage.

Structure of bacteriophage

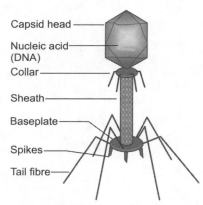

Figure 5.5: Bacteriophage

- **Lytic Cycle:** The process by which a bacteriophage attacks, multiplies and kills a bacterial cell is called as lytic cycle. The bacterial cell which is attacked is called as host cell.

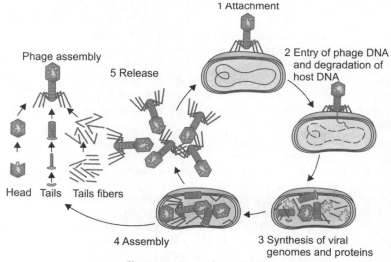

Figure 5.6: Steps of transduction

Steps of Transduction

- **Step 1:** The bacteriophage attacks the host bacterial cell (called as donor cell) and injects its DNA.

- **Step 2:** The bacteriophage DNA then makes a special type of enzyme that degrades (or break down) the host DNA.
- **Step 3:** New bacteriophage particles are synthesized each having bacteriophage DNA (usual bacteriophage) and few with host's (or donor's) DNA (unusual bacteriophage). Such unusual bacteriophage is called as a transducing phage.
- **Step 4:** The transducing phage attacks another bacterial cell (also called as recipient cell) and injects donor's DNA.
- **Step 5:** Donor's DNA is then incorporated into recipient's chromosome by recombination. After this the recipient cell is called as transduced cell.

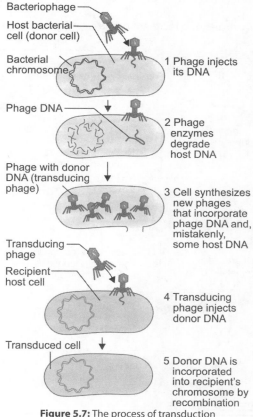

Figure 5.7: The process of transduction

Transformation

Definition: Transformation is a process in which bacteria take-up DNA from the outside environment and integrates into its chromosome.

Steps of Transformation

- Naked DNA fragments from one bacterium (donor) released during cell lysis (when cell bursts) bind to the cell wall of another bacterium (recipient).
- The recipient bacterium must be competent which means that it has structures on its cell wall that can bind DNA and take it up into it.
- The DNA that has been brought in can then incorporate itself into the recipient.
- After this process, the recipient cell is called as transformed cell.

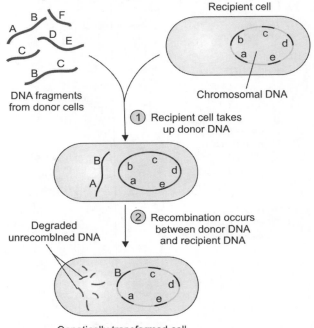

Figure 5.8: Transformation in bacteria

■ POSSIBLE QUESTIONS

1. **What is reproduction? Discuss various types of Asexual reproduction carried out by microorganisms.**
2. **Write an essay on various types of Sexual reproduction seen in Microorganisms.**

3. What is sexual reproduction? How is it different from asexual reproduction? Write a short note on transduction.
4. **Write Short Notes:**
    - Binary fission
    - Budding
    - Conidia
    - Cyst
    - Sporulation
    - Endospore
    - Bacteriophage
    - Lytic cycle
    - Transduction
    - Conjugation
    - Transformation
    - Zoospores

Chapter

6

Growth and Nutrition of Microorganisms

■ WHAT IS GROWTH IN MICROORGANISMS?

Growth is an essential characteristic of living organisms. For example a human baby grows to become an adult, a small plant grows to become a huge tree, etc. But how do microorganisms grow? They are always microscopic after all. Growth of microorganisms always means increase in their population (i.e. cell number). In bacteria, this happens by the process of binary fission.

■ CLASSIFICATION OF MICROORGANISMS ON NUTRITION BASIS

All living organisms require a source of energy. Depending on this, the microbes can be classified as;

- Phototrophs: organisms that use radiant energy (light) are called phototrophs. Example, Cyanobacteria.
- Chemotrophs: microorganisms that obtain energy by Oxidation of electron donors in their environment. These molecules can be organic or inorganic. Example, *Nitrobacter*.
- Lithotrophs- organisms that oxidize inorganic compounds are called lithotrophs. Example, Purple sulfur bacteria.

The carbon requirements of organisms must be met by organic carbon (a chemical compound with a carbon-hydrogen bond) or by CO_2.

- Heterotrophs: Organisms that use organic carbon are called as heterotrophs. Example, *E. coli.*
- Autotrophs: organisms that use CO_2 as a sole source of carbon for growth are called **autotrophs**. Example, Green bacteria.

Table 6.1. Major nutritional types of prokaryotes

Nutritional Type	Energy Source	Carbon Source	Examples
Photoautotrophs	Light	CO_2	Cyanobacteria, some purple and green bacteria
Photohetero-trophs	Light	Organic Compounds	Some purple and green bacteria
Chemoautotrophs			
or Lithotrophs (Lithoautotrophs)	Inorganic compounds, e.g. H_2, NH_3, NO_2, H_2S	CO_2	A few bacteria and many Archaea
Chemohetero-trophs or Hetero-trophs	Organic compounds	Organic Compounds	Most bacteria, some Archaea

■ FACTORS AFFECTING MICROBIAL GROWTH

(a) Nutrition

- Nutrients that are acquired from the environment are used for growth by microorganisms.
- These nutrients are classified as macro and microelements;

The Macroelements

- Macroelements consist of C, H, O, N, S, P, K, Mg, Fe, Ca, Mn, Zn, Co, Cu, and Mo. These elements are found in the form of water, inorganic ions, small molecules and macromolecules which serve either a structural or functional role in cells.

Table 6.2. Major elements, their sources and functions in bacterial cells

Elements	% of dry weight	Sources	Functions
Carbon	50	Organic compounds or CO_2	Main constituent of cellular material
Oxygen	20	H_2O, Organic compounds, CO_2, and O_2	Constituent of cell material and cell water; O_2 is electron acceptor in aerobic respiration
Nitrogen	14	NH_3, NO_3, organic compounds, N_2	Constituent of Amino acids, Nucleic acids Nucleotides and coenzymes

Cont...

Cont...

Elements	% of dry weight	Sources	Functions
Hydrogen	8	H_2O, organic compounds, H_2	Main constituent of organic compounds and cell water
Phosphorus	3	Inorganic phosphates (PO_4)	Constituent of nucleic acids, nucleotides, phospholipids, LPS, teichoic acids
Sulphur	1	SO_4, H_2S, So, organic Sulphur compounds	Constituent of cysteine, methionine, glutathione, several coenzymes
Potassium	1	Potassium salts	Main cellular inorganic cation and cofactor for certain enzymes
Magnesium	0.5	Magnesium salts	Inorganic cellular cation, cofactor for certain enzymatic reactions
Calcium	0.5	Calcium salts	Inorganic cellular cation, cofactor for certain enzymes and a component of endospores
Iron	0.2	Iron salts	Component of cytochromes and certain nonheme iron-proteins and a cofactor for some enzymatic reactions

Microelements

Microelements or trace elements are metal ions required by certain cells in small amounts. Example, Mn, Co, Zn, Cu and Mo.

(b) Oxygen Requirement

Microorganisms can be classified on the basis of oxygen requirement:
- Aerobes: They need oxygen for growth. Example, *Streptococci*, *Staphylococcus*.
- Anaerobe: they don't need oxygen for growth. Example, *Clostridium*
- Obligate aerobes: They absolutely require O_2 for growth. Example *Mycobacterium tuberculosis* and *Nocardia asteroides*.
- Obligate anaerobes (occasionally called aerophobes) They do not need O_2 at all. In fact, O_2 is poisonous to them. Examples, Actinomyces, Bacteroides, Fusobacterium.
- Facultative anaerobes: They can switch between aerobic and anaerobic states. Example, *Escherichia coli (E. coli)*.

- Aerotolerant anaerobes: They are insensitive to the presence of O_2. Example, *Clostridium intestinale*.
- Microaerophilic: They need little amount of oxygen for growth. Example- *Campylobacter jejuni*.

Table 6.3: Terms used to describe O_2 relations of microorganisms

Organism	Obligate aerobe	Facultative anaerobe	Obligate anaerobe	Aero-tolereant anaerobe	Microaero-phile
Effort of oxygen on oxygen	Oxygen required. Only can survive in aerobic conditions. Dies if oxygen is absent.	Growth in presence of oxygen, both aerobic and anaerobic.	Oxygen not required, only can surive in anaerobic conditions. Dies if oxygen is present.	Do not care if oxygen is present or absent. Just do not use the oxygen present.	Low oxygen concentration allowed for growth only.
Examples	*Mycobacterium*	*Streptococcus, Staphylococcus, Enterobacteriaceae*	*Clostridium*	*Lactobacillus*	*Neisseria gonorrhoeae*

(c) pH

- The pH is the hydrogen ion concentration $[H^+]$, of a liquid. It varies from 0.5–10.5 and above. If a liquid has a pH in the range 0.5–6 then it is considered as acidic, 7 is neutral (neither acidic nor alkaline) and 7 above is considered as alkaline or basic.

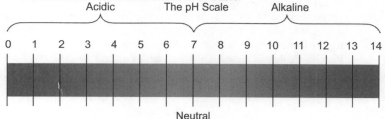

Figure 6.1: The pH scale

- The range of pH over which a microorganism grows is defined by **three cardinal points: minimum pH** below which organisms cannot grow, maximum pH, above which organisms cannot grow and **optimum pH** at which the organism grows the best.
- Depending on the optimum pH requirement, microorganisms can be classified as

Acidophiles: Microorganisms which grow at an optimum pH well between 0.5-6 are called **acidophiles**. Example, *Thiobacillus, Sulfolobus*.

- Neutrophiles: Those which grow the best at neutral pH (pH 7) are called neutrophiles. Example, Soil bacteria and yeasts.
- Alkaliphiles: Those that grow best under alkaline conditions (pH above 7) are called alkaliphiles. Example, *Clostridium, Bacillus.*

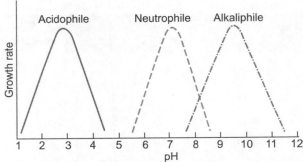

Figure 6.2: Growth rate vs pH for three environmental classes of microorganisms

(d) Temperature

Depending upon the temperature requirement, microorganisms can be categorized as:

- Mesophile: Microorganisms which can grow best (optimum temperature) at temperature near 37°C (the body temperature of human beings) are called **mesophiles**. Example, *Staphylococcus aureus, Salmonella, Listeria,* etc.
- Thermophiles: Microorganisms which can grow best at a temperature between about 45° and 70° are called **thermophiles**. Example, *Alicyclobacillus.*
- Hyperthermophiles: Some thermophiles can even grow at a temperature of 80°C or as high as 115°C. They are called as **hyperthermophiles**. Example, *Methanopyrus.*
- Psychrophiles- The cold-loving microorganisms are **psychrophiles**. They have the ability to grow at 0°C. Example, *Psychrobacter.*

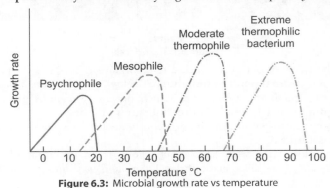

Figure 6.3: Microbial growth rate vs temperature

(e) Solute and Water Availability

For microorganisms solute can be salt (NaCl) or sugar. Depending on salt and water availability, the Microorganisms could be categorized as follows;

- Halophiles: These are microorganisms that require sodium chloride (NaCl), the common salt, for growth. Example- Halobacteria. They are of following types;
  - **Mild halophiles** require 1-6% salt.
  - **Moderate halophiles** require 6-15% salt.
  - **Extreme halophiles** that require 15-30% salt.
- Halotolerant: These are microorganisms that are able to grow at moderate salt concentrations even though they grow best in absence of NaCl. Example, *Cyanobacteria.*
- Osmophiles: Microorganisms that are able to live in environments high in sugar. Example, *Enterobacter aerogenes, Micrococcus.*
- Xerophiles: Microorganisms which live in dry environment (made dry by lack of water). Example, *Trichosporonoides.*

■ CALCULATION OF MICROBIAL GROWTH

- Bacteria can increase their number by carrying out the process of binary fission. Suppose there is one bacterial cell. It takes 2 minutes to divide into two daughter cells through binary fission. So when one bacterial cell divides to form two we say one generation is over. The time taken by the bacterial cell to double its number is called as its generation time. For example, like in the above case the generation time is 2 minutes.

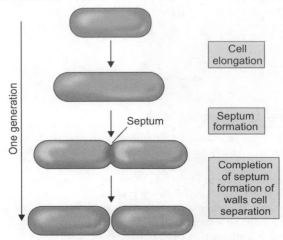

Figure 6.4: Formation of one generation in bacteria

- The generation time can mathematically be expressed as;

g = t/n
t is the duration of exponential growth.
n is the number of generations during the period of exponential growth.

Table 6.4: Generation times for some common bacteria

Bacterium	Generation Time (minutes)
Escherichia coli	17
Bacillus megaterium	25
Streptococcus lactis	26
Streptococcus lactis	48
Staphylococcus aureus	27–30
Lactobacillus acidophilus	66–87
Rhizobium japonicum	344–461
Mycobacterium tuberculosis	792–932
Treponema pallidum	1980

The growth pattern of bacteria is exponential in nature. This means under favourable conditions, a growing bacterial population doubles at regular intervals. Growth is by geometric progression: 1, 2, 4, 8, etc. or 20, 21, 22, 23.........2n (where n = the number of generations). This is called **exponential growth**.

A relationship exists between the initial and final number of bacterial cell present. This can be presented as follows;

$N = N_0 2^n$
N is the final cell number.
N_0 is the initial cell number.
n is the number of generations during the period of exponential growth.

■ MICROBIAL GROWTH CYCLE

The entire series of events that include birth, maturation and death of microorganisms could be put together to form the microbial growth cycle.

The microbial growth cycle is represented by microbial growth curve on a graph sheet. This has following phases:
- **Lag phase:** The population of microorganisms remains the same as bacteria become accustomed to their new environment.
- **Logarithmic phase (log phase):** Bacterial growth occurs at its optimal level and the population doubles rapidly.

- **Stationary phase:** The reproduction of bacterial cells is offset by their death and the population reaches a plateau. The reasons for bacterial death include accumulation of waste, lack of nutrients and unfavourable environmental conditions that may have developed.
- **Decline phase (Death Phase):** If the conditions are not changed, the population will enter its decline or death phase. The bacteria die off rapidly, the curve turns downward and the last cell in the population soon dies.

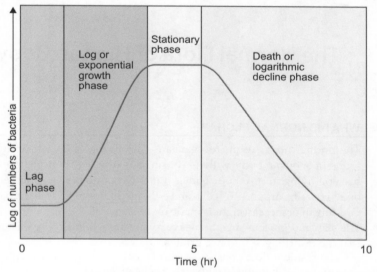

Figure 6.5: Growth curve of bacteria

■ POSSIBLE QUESTIONS

1. What is microbial growth? What are the factors affecting the bacterial growth?
2. Discuss in detail about different phases of microbial growth curve.
3. Write Short Notes:
   - Phototroph
   - Chemotroph
   - Lithotroph
   - Macronutrients and Micronutrients
   - Psychrophiles
   - Mesophiles
   - Thermophiles
   - Halophiles
   - Aerobe and anaerobe
   - Microbial growth curve

Chapter

7

The Normal Flora of Human Body

■ WHAT IS NORMAL FLORA?

- The normal flora are microorganisms (mostly bacteria) which are found in or on our body without causing any disease. There are more bacteria living in or on our bodies, than that of our cells. A human body contains around 10^{13} cells and is home to around 10^{14} bacteria. One fourth of faecal weight is made up of bacteria!
- The skin and mucous membranes carry a variety of microorganisms that can be arranged into two groups:
  - The resident flora consists of permanent microorganisms which are regularly found in a given area at a given age.
  - The transient flora consists of nonpathogenic or pathogenic microorganisms that stay on the skin or mucous membranes for hours, days, or weeks. They come from the environment, do not produce disease and do not stay permanently on the surface.

■ DISTRIBUTION OF NORMAL FLORA IN THE BODY

The most common sites of body inhabited by normal flora are the skin, eye, mouth, upper respiratory, gastrointestinal and urogenital tracts.

Normal microbiota of the conjunctiva
1. Coagulase-nagative *Staphylococci*
2. *Haemophilus* spp.
3. *Staphylococcus aureus*
4. *Streptococci* (various species)

Normal microbiota of the outer ear
1. Coagulase-nagative
   Staphylococci
2. *Diphtheroids*
3. *Pseudomonas* spp.
4. *Enterobacteriaceae*
   (Peptostreptococcus)

Normal microbiota of
the stomach
1. *Streptococcus*
2. *Staphylococcus*
3. *Lactobacillus*
4. *Peptostreptococcus*

Normal microbiota of
the skin
1. Coagulase-nagative
   Staphylococci
2. *Diphtheroids* (including
   Propionibacterium acnes)
3. *Staphylococcus aureus*
4. *Streptococci* (various species)
5. *Bacillus* spp.
6. *Malassezia furfur*
7. *Candida* spp.
8. *Mycobacterium* spp.
   (occasionally)

Normal microbiota of the urethra
1. Coagulase-nagative *Staphylococci*
2. *Diphtheroids*
3. *Streptococci* (various species)
4. *Mycobacterium* spp.
5. *Bacteroides* spp. and
   Fusobacterium spp.
6. *Peptostreptococcus* spp.

Normal microbiota of the vagina
1. *Lactobacillus* spp.
2. *Peptostreptococcus* spp.
3. *Diphtheroids*
4. *Streptococci* (various)
5. *Clostridium* spp.
6. *Bacteroides* spp.
7. *Candida* spp.
8. *Gardnerella vaginalis*

Normal microbiota of the nose
1. Coagulase-negative
   Staphylococci
2. *Viridans streptococci*
3. *Staphylococcus aureus*
4. *Neisseria* spp.
5. *Haemophilus* spp.
6. *Streptococcus pneumoniae*

Normal microbiota of the
mouth and oropharynx
1. *Viridians streptococci*
2. Coagulase-negative
   Staphylococci
3. *Veillonella* spp.
4. *Fusobacterium* spp.
5. *Treponema* spp.
6. *Porphyromonas* spp.
   and *Prevotella* spp.
7. *Neisseria* spp. and
   Branhamella catarrhalis
8. *Streptococcus pneumoniae*
9. Beta-hemolytic
   Streptococci (not group A)
10. *Candida* spp.
11. *Haemophilus* spp.
12. *Diphtheroids*
13. *Actinomyces* spp.
14. *Ekenella corrodens*
15. *Staphylococcus aureus*

Normal microbiota of the
small intestine
1. *Lactobacillus* spp.
2. *Bacteroides* spp.
3. *Clostridium* spp.
4. *Mycobacterium* spp.
5. *Enterococci*
6. *Enterobacteriaceae*

Normal microbiota of the large
intestine
1. *Bacteroides* spp.
2. *Fusobacterium* spp.
3. *Clostridium* spp.
4. *Peptostreptococcus* spp.
5. *Escherichia coli*
6. *Klebsiella* spp.
7. *Proteus* spp.
8. *Lactobacillus* spp.
9. *Enterococci*
10. *Streptococci* (various species)
11. *Pseudomonas* spp.
12. *Acinetobacter* spp.
13. Coagulase-negative *Staphylococci*
14. *Staphylococcus aureus*
15. *Mycobacterium* spp.
16. *Actinomyces* spp.

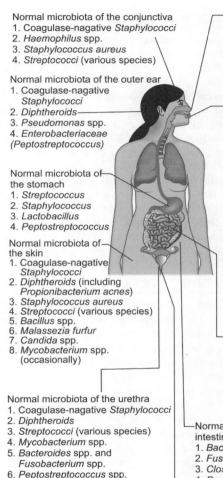

Figure 7.1: Normal flora of human body

■ BENEFICIAL FUNCTIONS OF NORMAL FLORA

- **The normal flora synthesize and excrete vitamins** in excess of their own needs which can be absorbed as nutrients by their host. For example, in humans, enteric bacteria secrete Vitamin K and Vitamin B12, and Lactic acid bacteria produce certain B-vitamins.
- **The normal flora prevent spreading of pathogens by competing for** attachment sites or for getting essential nutrients.
- **The normal flora may antagonize (act against) other bacteria** through production of substances which inhibit or kill pathogenic bacteria. For example the intestinal bacteria produce a variety of substances such as bacteriocins, which inhibit or kill other bacteria.
- **The normal flora stimulates development of certain tissues.** For example, the caecum of germ-free animals is enlarged, thin-walled and fluid-filled compared to that in other animals.
- **The normal flora stimulates production of natural antibodies.** Since normal flora behave as antigens in an animal, they induce an immunological response, in particular, an antibody-mediated immune (AMI) response.

■ HARMFUL EFFECTS OF NORMAL FLORA

- **Bacterial synergism** between a member of normal flora and a potential pathogen. This means one organism is helping another to grow or survive. There are examples of a member of the normal flora supplying vitamin or some other growth factor that a pathogen needs in order to grow. This is called **cross-feeding** between microbes. Another example of synergism occurs during treatment of **"staph-protected infections"** when a penicillin-resistant *Staphylococcus* that is a component of the normal flora shares its drug resistance with pathogens that are otherwise susceptible to the drug.
- **Competition for nutrients** Bacteria in the gastrointestinal tract must absorb some of the host's nutrients for their own needs.
- Minute amounts of bacterial toxins (e.g. endotoxin) may be found in the circulation. Of course, it is these small amounts of bacterial antigen that stimulate the formation of natural antibodies.
- **The normal flora may be agents of disease.** Members of normal flora may cause **endogenous disease** if they reach a site or tissue where they cannot be restricted or tolerated by the host defenses.
- Some pathogens of humans that are members of normal flora may also rely on their host for transfer to other individuals where they can produce disease. This includes pathogens that colonize the upper respiratory tract such as *Neisseria meningitidis, Streptococcus pneumoniae, Haemophilus influenzae and Staphylococcus aureus and potential pathogens such as E. coli, Salmonella or Clostridium* in the gastrointestinal tract.

■ POSSIBLE QUESTIONS

1. Write an essay on the normal flora of human body.
2. Explain about normal flora of human body. What are its benefits and harmful effects?

Chapter

8

Pathogenic Microorganisms

■ INTRODUCTION

- Microorganisms can be found at every place and in close association with every type of multicellular organism. They grow on healthy human body by billions as harmless normal flora. All microoraganisms do not cause disease. Those relatively few species of microorganisms that are harmful to humans by causing diseases are called as pathogens.
- Most infectious disease started by colonization (the establishment of multiplying microorganisms on the skin or mucous membranes) Microbial colonization may result in:

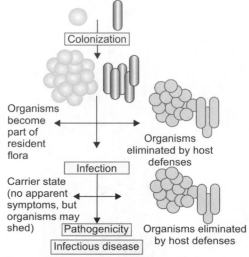

Figure 8.1: Some possible outcomes following exposure of microorganisms

- elimination (or removal) of microorganism without affecting the host
- infection in which the an organisms multiply and cause the host to react
- a short period or prolonged carrier state.

Infectious disease occurs when an organism causes tissue damage and affecting body function.

■ PATHOGENIC AND NON-PATHOGENIC MICROORGANISMS

Any organism or agent that produces a disease is called as a a pathogen (Greek *patho*, disease, and *gennan*, to produce). Its ability to cause disease is called pathogenicity. Microorganisms which do not cause any disease are called as non-pathogenic microorganisms. Followings are types of pathogen;

- **Primary pathogen** is any organism that causes disease in a healthy host by direct interaction.
- **Opportunistic pathogen** is an organism that is either normally free-living or a part of the host's normal flora but which may adopt a pathogenic role under certain circumstances such as when the immune system is weak.
- Host is a living organism on which the pathogen grow and cause disease. Followings are the types of hosts:
  - **Final host:** The host on or in which the parasitic organism either attains sexual maturity or reproduces.
  - **Intermediate host:** A host that serves as a temporary but essential environment for some stages of development.
  - **Transfer host:** This is not necessary for completion of the organism's life cycle but is used as a vehicle for reaching a final host.
  - **Reservoir host:** A host infected with a parasitic organism that also can infect humans.

Table 8.1: Categorization of Parasitic organisms and agents by size

Discipline	Parasitic Group		Approximate Size
Virology	Prions	} Agents	350 k Da
	Viroids	} 25–400 nm	130 k Da
	Viruses		
Bacteriology	Chlamydiac		0.2–1.5 mm
	Mycoplasmas		0.3–0.8 mm
	Rickettsias		0.5–2 mm
	Other bacteria		
		Microorganisms (Microbiota)	

Cont...

Cont...

Discipline		Parasitic Group		Approxi-mate Size
Mycology		Fungi		3-15 mm diameter (hyphae)
Protozoology		Protozoa		1-150 mm
Helminthology	} Parasitology	Nematodes Platyhel-minthes (cestodes, trematodes)	} Parasites	3 mm – 30 cm 1 mm – 10 m
Entomology		Ticks and miltes		15 mm
Zoology		Horsehair worms Mesozoa Leeches	} Ectoparasites	10-20 cm Up to 100 cm 1-5 cm

■ HOST-PARASITE RELATIONSHIP

- If an organism either harms or lives at the expense of another organism (the host) then the former an organism is called as a parasitic an organism and the relationship is called parasitism. The parasitic organism is usually smaller and is dependent on the host. There are many parasitic agents or organisms among the viruses, bacteria, fungi, plants and animals.
- There are two types of parasites which are:
  - Ectoparasite: If an organism lives on the surface of its host.
  - Endoparasite: If it lives internally inside the body of the host.

When a parasite is growing and multiplying within or on a host, the host is said to have an infection. An infection may or may not result in disease. An infectious disease is any change from a state of health in which part or all of the host body is not capable of carrying on its normal functions due to the presence of an organism or its products.

- The term virulence refers to the degree or intensity of pathogenicity of pathogen. It is determined by three characteristics of the pathogen:
  - Invasiveness: The ability of an organism to spread to adjacent or other tissues.
  - Infectivity: The ability of an organism to establish a point of infection.
  - Pathogenic potential: This refers to the degree that the pathogen causes damage. A major aspect of pathogenic potential is toxigenicity.

- Toxigenicity is pathogen's ability to produce toxins. Toxins are chemical substances that will damage the host and produce disease.

The outcome of most host-parasite relationships is dependent on three main factors:
- – The number of organisms present in or on the host
- – The virulence of an organism
- – The host's defenses or degree of resistance.

Table 8.2: Terms used to describe infection

Type	Definition
Abscess	A localize infection with collection of pus surrounded by an inflamed area
Acute	Short but serve course
Bacteremia	Presence of viable bacteria in the blood
Chronic	Persists over a long time
Covert	Subclinical, no symptoms
Cross	Transmitted between hots infected with different organisms
Focal	Exists in circumscribed areas
Fulminating	Infectious agent multiplies with great intensity
Latrogenic	Caused as a result of health care
Latent	Persists in tissues for long periods, during most of which there are no symptoms
Localized	Restricted to a limited region or to none or more anatomical areas
Mixed	More than one organism present simultaneously
Nosocomial	Develops during a stay at a hospital or other clinical care facility
Opportunistic	Due to an agent that does not harm a healthy host but takes advantage of an unhealthy one
Overt	Symptomatic
Phytogenic	Caused by plant pathogens
Primary	First infection that often allows other organisms to appear on the scene
Pyogenic	Result in pus formation
Secondary	Caused by an organism following an initial or primary infection
Sepsis	The condition resulting from the presence of bacteria or their toxins in blood or tissues; the presence of pathogens or their toxins in the blood or other tissues

Cont...

Cont...

Type	Definition
	Systemic response to infection; this systemic response is manifested by two or more of the following conditions as a result of infection: temperature, >38°C or <36°C; heart rate, >90 beats per min; respiratory rate, >20 breaths per min, or pCO_2, <32 mm Hg; leukocyte count, > 12000 cells per ml^3. Or >10% immature (band) forms
Septicemia	Blood poisoning associated with persistence of pathogenic organisms or their toxins in the blood
Septic shock	Sepsis with hypotension despite adequate fluid resuscitation, along with the presence of perfusion abnormalities that may include but are not limited to, lactic acidosis, oliguria, or an acute alteration in mental status
Severe sepsis	Sepsis is associated with organ dysfunction, hypoperfusion, or hypotension; hypoperfusion and perfusion abnormalities that may include; but are not limited to, lactic acidosis, oliguria, or an acute alteration in mental status
Sporadic	Occurs occasionally
Subclinical (inapparent or convert)	No detectable symptoms or manifestations,
Toxemia	Condition arising from toxins in the blood
Zoonosis	Caused by a parasitic organism that is normally found in animals orther than humans

■ MECHANISM OF INFECTIOUS PROCESS

- **Entry into the host:** The first step of infectious process is the entry of microorganism into the host by one of several ports: via respiratory, gastrointestinal (GI), urogenital tract or through skin that has been cut, punctured, or burnt. Once entry is achieved, the pathogen must overcome diverse host immune system before it can establish itself. These include
  - Phagocytosis
  - The acidic environments of stomach and urogenital tract
  - Various hydrolytic and proteolytic enzymes found in saliva, stomach and small intestine.
- Adherence of microorganism to host cells: Various bacteria follow different mechanisms to adhere (attach) to the surface of host cells. For example, *Escherichia coli* use pili whereas Group A *Streptococci* uses its fimbriae to adhere to the surface of the host cells. In each case, adherence enhances virulence by preventing bacteria from being carried away by mucous or washed from organs with significant fluid flow, such as the urinary and the GI tracts.

- Invasion of the host: Invasive bacteria are those that can enter host cells or penetrate mucosal surfaces, spreading from the initial site of infection. Invasiveness is facilitated by several bacterial enzymes, the most notable of which are collagenase and hyaluronidase.

- Propagation of the Microorganism: Once the pathogen has entered the host it will start to propagate (or multiply) very fast in order to increase its number.

- Damage to host cell: While propagating itself in the host cell, microorganisms can damage the host cell by producing toxins. They are of two types:

  - Exotoxins: These are toxins which are produced and released by the pathogenic bacteria at the site of their multiplication. For example, diphtheria toxin. Exotoxins are proteins secreted by both Gram-positive and Gram-negative bacteria.

  - Endotoxins: These are not released out but instead is part of the cell walls of Gram-negative bacteria. For Example LPS, layer of Gram-negative bacteria.

Table 8.3: Characteristics of bacterial endotoxins and classic exotoxin

PROPERTY	ENDOTOXIN	EXOTOXIN
CHEMICAL NATURE	Lipopolysaccharide (mw = 10kDa)	Protein (mw = 50-1000kDa)
RELATIONSHIP TO CELL	Part of outer membrane	Extracellular, diffusible
DENATURED BY BOILING	No	Usually
ANTIGENIC	Yes	Yes
FORM TOXOID	No	Yes
POTENCY	Relatively low (>100 µg)	Relatively high (1 µg)
SPECIFICITY	Low degree	High degree
ENZYMATIC ACTIVITY	No	Often
PYROGENICITY	Yes	Occasionally

Damage of the host cell is also possible due to host immune response.

- Progression or resolution of disease: If the pathogen is not removed by immune system then the disease is established. If the pathogen fails to multiply then there is no disease.

1. Entry into the host, with evasion of host primary defenses

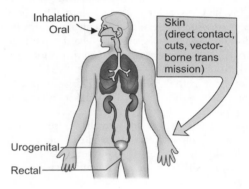

Inhalation
Oral
Skin (direct contact, cuts, vector-borne trans mission)
Urogenital
Rectal

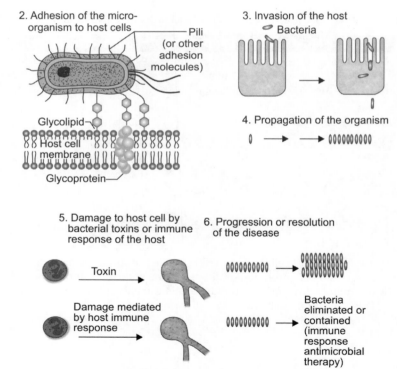

2. Adhesion of the micro-organism to host cells
Pili (or other adhesion molecules)
Glycolipid
Host cell membrane
Glycoprotein

3. Invasion of the host
Bacteria

4. Propagation of the organism

5. Damage to host cell by bacterial toxins or immune response of the host
Toxin
Damage mediated by host immune response

6. Progression or resolution of the disease

Bacteria eliminated or contained (immune response antimicrobial therapy)

Figure 8.2: Mechanism of infectious process

■ POSSIBLE QUESTIONS

1. What are pathogenic microorganisms? How are they different from non-pathogenic microorganisms?
2. Write an essay on host-parasite relationship.
3. What is infection? Give a detailed account of the mechanism of infectious process.
4. Write Short Notes:
   - Pathogen
   - Parasite
   - Pathogenicity
   - Virulence
   - Host
   - Infection
   - Invasiveness
   - Endotoxin and Exotoxins
   - Infectivity

Chapter
9

Diseases Caused by Microorganisms

■ INTRODUCTION

A few harmful microbes for example, less than 1% of bacteria, can invade our body (the host) and make us ill. They are called as pathogenic microorganisms.

Pathogens establish infection and damage tissues by any of three mechanisms:

- They can contact or enter host cells and directly cause of death cells.
- They may release toxins that kill cells at a distance, release enzymes that degrade tissue components or damage blood vessels .
- They can induce host immune responses that although directed against the invader(pathogen), cause additional tissue damage.

■ COMMON DISEASES CAUSED BY BACTERIA (FIG. 9.1 AND TABLE 9.1)

Millions of bacteria normally live on the skin, in the intestines and on genitalia. The vast majority of bacteria do not cause disease. Many bacteria are actually helpful and even necessary for good health.

These bacteria are sometimes referred to as "good bacteria" or "healthy bacteria."

Harmful bacteria that cause bacterial infections and diseases are called pathogenic bacteria. Bacterial diseases occur when pathogenic bacteria get into the body, begin to reproduce and crowd out healthy bacteria, or to grow in tissues that are normally sterile. Harmful bacteria may also emit toxins that damage the body. Common pathogenic bacteria and the types of bacterial diseases they cause include:

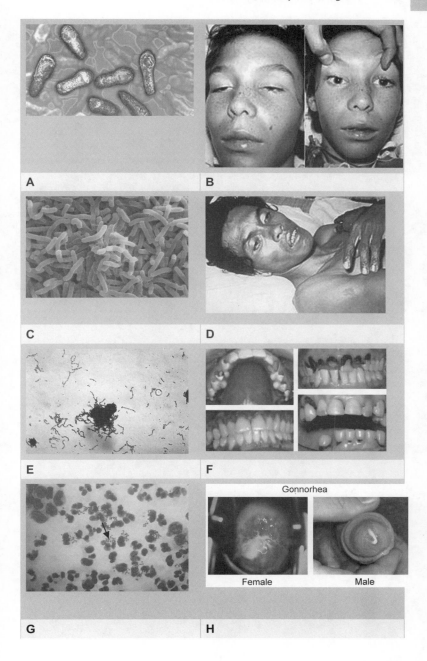

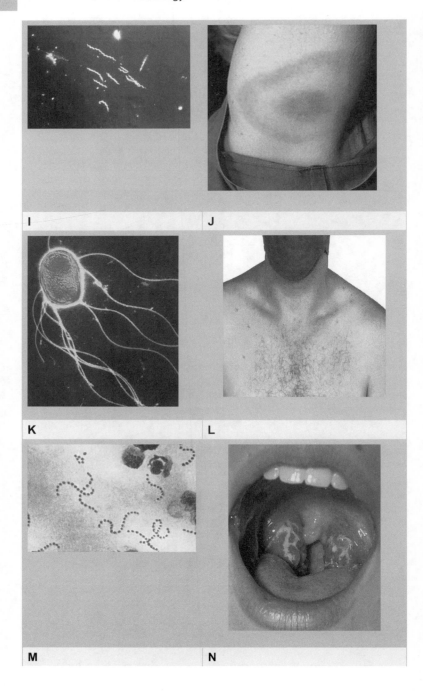

I

J

K

L

M

N

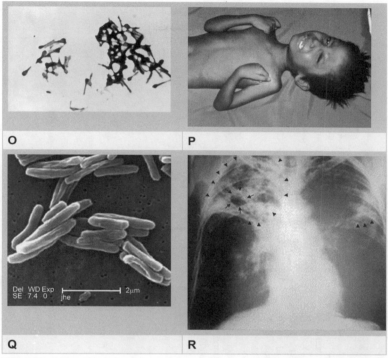

Figures 9.1 (A to R): Common Bacterial diseases of human beings. (A) *Clostridium botulinum*, causal organism of botulism, (B) A 14-year-old patient with botulism, (C) *Vibrio cholerae* causal organism of cholera, (D) A person with severe dehydration due to cholera, (E) *Streptococcus mutans*, causal organism of dental caries, (F) Dental caries, (G) *Neisseria gonorrhoeae*, causal organism of gonorrhoeae, (H) Gonorrhoeae in male and female, (I) *Borrelia burgdorferi*, causal organism of Lyme disease, (J) Classic bull's-eye appearance is also called erythema migrans, (K) *Salmonella typhi*, causal organism of typhoid (L) Rose spots on the chest of a patient with typhoid fever due to the bacterium *Salmonella*, (M) *Streptococcus pyogenes*, causal organism of streptococcal pharyngitis, (N) Streptococcal pharyngitis, (O) *Clostridium tetani*, causal organism of tetanus, (P) A child suffering from tetanus, (Q) *Mycobacterium tuberculosis*, causal organism of tuberculosis, (R) Chest X-ray of a person with advanced tuberculosis: Infection in both lungs is marked by white arrow-heads and the formation of a cavity is marked by black arrows. *(For color version see plates 1 to 3)*

Table 9.1: Common bacterial diseases

Diseases	Pathogenic Agent	Transmission	Symptoms	Target Body part	Treatment and prevention
Botulism	Clostridium botulinum	Improperly preserved foods	Difficulty swallowing/ speaking dry mouth. Facial weakness Burred vision. Trouble breathing Nausea, abdominal cramps	Nerves	The Patient is kept on a ventilator for weeks/months. Patient is treated with Antitoxin
Cholera	Vibrio cholerae	Contaminated water and food	Diarrhoea, vomiting, dehydration (loss of water). headache, stomach ache	Intestine	Antibiotics, Vaccination, Replace fluids intravenously, drinking boiled water
Dental Caries	Streptococcus mutants	Enter the mouth from environment	Presence of a small pit, or hole, in the tooth, Sensitivity to hot and cold food and beverages, Bad breath (halitosis), Bitter taste in the mouth, Swelling of the gums, Facial swelling with enlarged glands in the neck	Teeth	Amalgam filling. Prevented by Brushing, flossing and reducing the intake of refined and processed sugars
Gonorrhea	Neisseria gonorrhoeae	By sexual contact	In Women- Greenish yellow or whitish discharge from the vagina, Lower abdominal or pelvic pain, Burning when urinating, Conjunctivitis (red, itchy eyes), Bleeding between periods, Spotting after inter-course, Swelling of the vulva (vulvitis), Burning in the throat (due to oral sex), Swollen glands in the throat (due to oral sex)	Female reproductive system– vagina, fallopian tubes uterus etc. Male reproductive and encretory organs– Penis, Urethra, urinary canal	Effective antibiotic treatment is given prevention:- practice safer sex or no sex untill antibiotic treatment is completed follow up test must be done to ensure clearance of infection.

Cont...

Cont...

Diseases	Pathogenic Agent	Transmission	Symptoms	Target Body part	Treatment and prevention
			In Man- Greenish yellow or whitish discharge from the penis, Burning when urinating, Painful or swollen testicles,		
Lyme Disease	*Borrelia burgdorferi*	Tick bite	Fever, headache and fatigue. A rash occurs in 70–80% of infected persons at the site of the tick bite after a delay of 3-30 days (average is about 7 days), and may or may not appear as the well-publicized bull's-eye	Skin, joints, heart	Oral administration of doxycycline. Protective clothing Light-colored clothing makes the tick more easily visible before it attaches itself. People should use special care in handling and allowing outdoor pets inside homes because they can bring ticks into the house.
Salmonella Food Poisoning (Typhoid)	*Salmonella typhii*	Contaminated water and food	Rash, headache, fever, coughing, body ache, weakness	Intestine	Vaccination, Antibiotics, Drinking boiled water

Cont...

Cont...

Diseases	Pathogenic Agent	Transmission	Symptoms	Target Body part	Treatment and prevention
Throat infection	Streptococcus pyogenes	Sneezing, coughs or direct person to person contact	Sore throat, fever of greater than 38 °C (100 °F), tonsillar exudates (pus on the tonsils), and large cervical lymph nodes	Upper respiratory tract, blood, skin	Analgesics such as non-steroidal anti-inflammatory drugs (NSAIDs) and paracetamol (acetaminophen) help significantly in the management of pain associated with strep throat. To avoid getting strep throat, it is a good idea to avoid contact with anyone who has a strep infection. Wash hands when you meet someone with bacterial or viral illnesses. Do not share toothbrushes or eating and drinking utensils.
Tetanus	Clostridium tetani	Contaminated wounds	Headache, Jaw cramping, Sudden, involuntary muscle tightening – often in the stomach (muscle spasms), Painful muscle stiffness all over the body, Trouble swallowing, Jerking or staring (seizures), Fever and sweating, High blood pressure and fast heart rate.	Nerves at synapses	Can be treated with; • Tetanus immunoglobulin, also called tetanus antibodies or tetanus antitoxin • Metronidazole IV for 10 days • Diazepam There are three different types of tetanus vaccines. Diphtheria, tetanus, and pertussis (DTaP), Tdap (tetanus, diphtheria, and pertussis), Td (tetanus and diphtheria) vaccine.

■ COMMON DISEASES CAUSED BY VIRUSES (FIG. 9.2 AND TABLE 9.2)

Viral diseases are extremely widespread infections caused by viruses, a type of microorganism. There are many types of viruses that cause a wide variety of viral diseases. The most common type of viral disease is the common cold, which is caused by a viral infection of the upper respiratory tract (nose and throat). Other common viral diseases include:

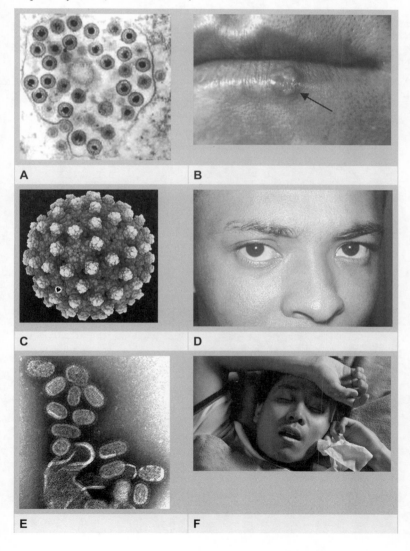

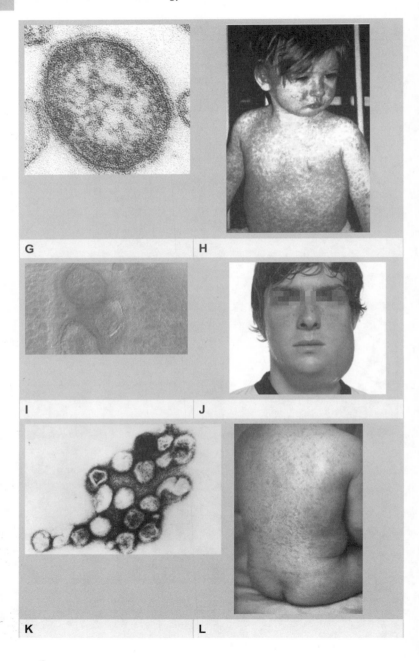

G

H

I

J

K

L

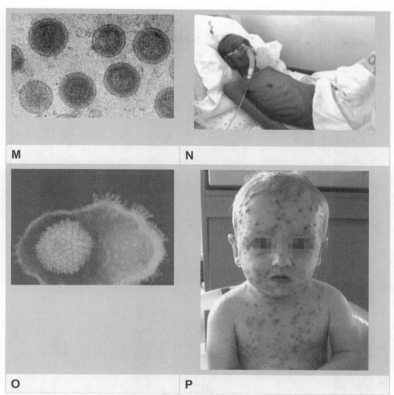

Figures 9.2 (A to P): Common Viral diseases in human beings. (A) Herpes virus, (B) Herpes labialis (blister) of the lower lip in a herpes patient, (C) Hepatitis A virus, (D) A case of jaundice caused by hepatitis A, (E) Influenza virus, (F) A patient suffering from Influenza, (G) Measles virus, (H) A patient suffering from measles, (I) Mumps virus, (J) A patient suffering from mumps, (K) Rubella Virus, (L) A patient suffering from Rubella (German fever), (M) Human Immunodeficiency virus (HIV), (N) A patient suffering from Acquired Immunodeficiency syndrome (AIDS), (O) *Varicella zoaster* virus, (P) A child suffering from small pox. *(For color version see plates 3 to 5)*

Table 9.2: Common viral diseases

Diseases	Pathogenic Agent	Transmission	Symptoms	Target Body part	Treatment and prevention
Tuberculosis	*Mycobacterium tuberculosis*	Person to person by coughs	A bad cough that lasts 3 weeks or longer, Pain in the chest, Coughing up blood or sputum (phlegm from deep inside the lungs), Weakness or fatigue, Weight loss, No appetite, Chills, Fever.	Lung, bones, other organs	Antibiotics used in the treatment of tuberculosis are Isoniazid, Rifampin (Rifadin, Rimactane), Ethambutol (Myambutol) and Pyrazinamide. Children are vaccinated with Bacille Calmette-Guerin (BCG) vaccine. For adults there is no vaccine.
Bacterial meningitis (Infection of sac around brain and spinal chord)	*Streptococcus pneumonia, Neisseria meningitides, Haemophilus influenzae* type b	Person to person through tiny droplets that are sent into the air during talking, laughing, coughing and sneezing. It can also spread by kissing, sharing eating utensils, and hand-to-hand contact.	Headache, sensitivity to light, neck stiffness, fever, loss of appetite, rashes, seizure, irritability in children and difficulty thinking clearly	Brain and Spinal Chord	Vaccination, Antibiotics such as ceftriaxone and vancomycin, Corticosteroids, drinking plenty of boiled water along with ample rest is advised. Prevention include- washing hands after contacting with patients
Herpes Simplex	Herpes virus hominis	Infections through droplets or infectious smears. Human may be carrier without symptoms	Fever blisters, severe weakness	Microscopically by demonstration of intranuclear inclusion bodies in cells from lesions	Aciclovir

Cont...

Cont...

Diseases	Pathogenic Agent	Transmission	Symptoms	Target Body part	Treatment and prevention
Hepatitis A	Hepatitis A Virus (HAV), Hepatitis epidemica	Oral infection by faeces, dirty hands or objects. Often transmitted by water, Active and passive vaccination in humans	Jaundice, fever, diarrhoea, rejection of food, seizures, itching, weakness, green-brown urine, often fatal	Detection of HAV in faeces; antibodies in serum	There is no specific treatment for hepatitis A. Sufferers are advised to rest, avoid fatty foods and alcohol (these may be poorly tolerated for some additional months during the recovery phase and cause minor relapses), eat a well-balanced diet, and stay hydrated
Influenza (Flu)	Influenza virus of humans; Coryza-Rhino viruses	Infection by humans (aerosol infection by sneezing) and in experiments	Sneezing, coughing, rhinitis, fever, headache, may affect respiratory organs	Viruses in respiratory tract	In case of secondary infections (pneumonia)
Rabies	Rabies Virus	Infection by bites, saliva of infected animals (carnivores, domestic animals) or by improper vaccination	Overexcitability, self-mutilation, inability to drink water, paralysis	Viruses in saliva, tears	Vaccination

Cont...

Cont...

Diseases	Pathogenic Agent	Transmission	Symptoms	Detection/Identification	Treatment
Measles	Measles Virus	It is spread when an infected person coughs, sneezes, or shares food or drinks. The measles virus can travel through the air.	Runny nose, high temperature, sore, red eyes, white spots inside mouth, red blotchy rash- it actually starts on the head and neck and spreads down the body, fever	Detected by viral culture or blood test	The measles vaccine protects against the illness. This vaccine is part of the MMR (measles, mumps, and rubella)
Mumps	Mumps Virus	Mumps is highly contagious. The virus is spread directly from one person to another via respiratory droplets, can also be transmitted via hand-to-mouth contact after touching infected pillows or bedsheets.	Swollen and painful salivary glands, flu like symptoms such as aches, pains and tiredness. Abdominal pain and headaches	Detected by clinical examination of parotid gland enlargement.	The Mumps vaccine protects against the illness. This vaccine is part of the MMR (measles, mumps, and rubella). Taking analgesics (acetaminophen, ibuprofen) and applying warm or cold packs to the swollen and inflamed salivary gland region may be helpful.
Rubella (German Measles)	Rubella Virus	It can spread when an infected person coughs or sneezes, or it can spread by direct contact with an infected person's respiratory secretions, such as mucus. It can also be transmitted from a pregnant woman to her unborn child via the bloodstream.	Rash that starts on face and spreads to the rest of the body, swollen glands behind ears and possibly in other parts of the body, mild fever, cold, cough, sore throat and red eyes.	Viral rashes are observed. Virus culture or a blood test can detect the presence of different types of rubella antibodies in your blood. These antibodies indicate whether the patient had a recent or past infection or a rubella vaccine.	No treatment will shorten the course of rubella infection, and symptoms are so mild that treatment usually isn't necessary. The rubella vaccine protects against the illness. This vaccine is part of the MMR (measles, mumps, and rubella).

Cont...

Cont...

Diseases	Pathogenic Agent	Transmission	Symptoms	Detection/ Identification	Treatment
AIDS	Human Immunodeficiency Virus (HIV)	From infected person via blood transfusion, semen (unprotected sex), use of infected needles, new born may acquire HIV from infected mother also.	Infected individuals have a flu-like illness within month or two after exposure to the virus, with fever, headache, tiredness, and enlarged lymph nodes (glands of the immune system). These symptoms usually disappear within a week to a month and are often mistaken for those of other viral infections. During this period, people are very infectious, and HIV is present in large quantities in blood, semen, and vaginal fluids. More severe HIV symptoms—such as profound and unexplained fatigue, rapid weight loss, frequent fevers, or profuse night sweats—may not appear for 10 years or more after HIV first enters the body in adults, or within two years in children born with HIV infection.	By testing blood for the presence of antibodies (disease-fighting proteins) to HIV	Since there is no accurate medication for HIV combined antiviral drugs are given to the patients. Prevention- Because there is no cure or vaccine to prevent HIV, the only way people can prevent infection from the virus is to avoid high-risk behaviors putting them at risk of infection, such as having unprotected sex or sharing needles.

Cont...

Cont...

Diseases	Pathogenic Agent	Transmission	Symptoms	Detection/Identification	Treatment
Viral Gastro-enteritis (Stomach Flu)	Rotavirus, Novovirus	Highly contagious, spreads through close contact with people who are infected, or through contaminated food or water.	Nausea, vomiting, loss of appetite, and watery diarrhea, fever and body aches, chills, sweating, abdominal cramps and pain, etc.	A stool sample is tested for the type of virus or the doctor finds out illness is due to a parasitic or bacterial infection, if not then its viral.	The main focus of treatment is to prevent dehydration by drinking plenty of fluids and electrolytes. Proper rest and food should be taken in small amounts. In severe cases, hospitalization and intravenous fluids are necessary.
Chicken Pox	*Varicella-Zoster Virus*	Virus can spread easily from one person to another. It most often spreads through the respiratory tract, such as mucous membranes of the mouth and nose. One can get chickenpox through the air from an infected person's sneezing or coughing.	Fever, tired and sluggish, no appetite, headache, sore throat, itchy rash and red spots or blisters all over the body.	Diagnosis is usually done based on the rash looks	Prevention- Chickenpox Vaccination.

■ COMMON DISEASES CAUSED BY FUNGI (FIG. 9.3 AND TABLE 9.3)

Clinical categories of fungal infections

- Superficial/Cutaneous: infection of outer layer of skin by lipophilic or keratinolytic fungi, e.g. pityriasis, dermatophytosis
- Subcutaneous: infection of subcutaneous tissues from the painful implantation of the fungus into the skin, e.g. sporotrichosis
- Systemic:
  - **The true pathogenic fungi**— can cause disease even in immunocompetent hosts: histoplasmosis, coccidioidomycosis, blastomycosis
  - **The opportunistic fungi**— generally cause disease only in immunocompromised hosts: cryptococcosis, candidiasis, aspergillosis, mucormycosis

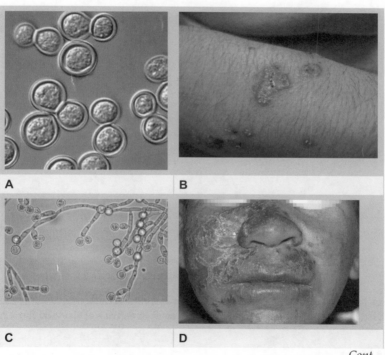

Cont...

Cont...

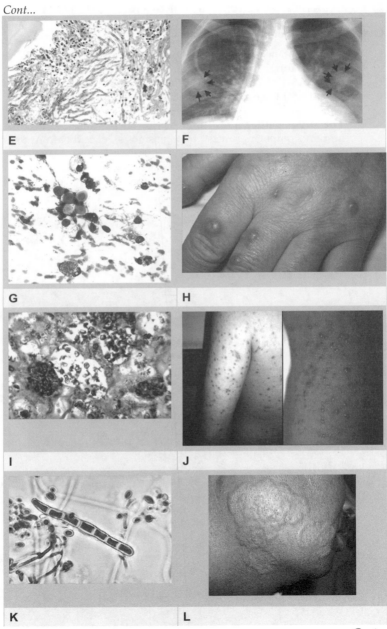

Cont...

Cont...

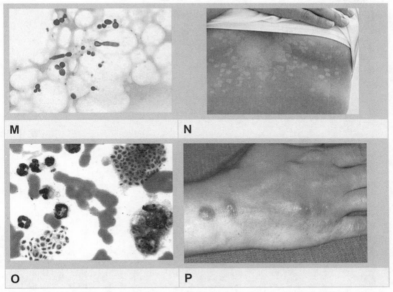

Figures 9.3 (A to P): Mycosis (A) *Blastomyces dermatitidis*, causal organism of Blastomycosis, (B) Blastomycosis, (C) *Candida albicans*, Causal organism of Candidiasis, (D) Candidiasis, (E) *Aspergillus* spp., causal organism of Aspergillosis, (F) Aspergillosis, (G) *Cryptococcus neoformans*, causal organism of Cryptococcosis, (H) Cryptococcosis, (I) *Histoplasma capsulatum*, causal organism of Histoplasmosis, (J) Colony of *Histoplasma capsulatum* inside the lungs of the patient suffering from Histoplasmosis, (K) *Tricophyton rubrum* (Dermatophyte), causal organisms of Dermatophytosis, (L) Dermatophytosis, (M) *Malassezia furfur*, causal organisms of Tinea versicolor (N) *Tinea versicolor*, (O) *Sporothrix schenckii*, causal organism of Sporotrichosis, (P) Sporotrichosis *(For color version see plates 5 to 8)*

Table 9.3: Common fungal infections (Mycosis)

Disease	Pathogenic Organisms	Pathogenesis	Symptoms	Diagnostic tests	Treatment
SUPERFICIAL FUNGAL INFECTIONS					
Dermatophytosis	Dermatophytes (Members of genera *Trichophyton*, *Microsporum and Epidermophyton*)	Spores on shed skin or hairs adhere to stratum corneum, germinate, invade. Organisms confined to stratum corneum, with surrounding inflammation penetrating deeper layers of skin	Can affect the skin on almost any area of the body, such as the scalp, legs, arms, feet groin, and nails. These infections are usually itchy. Redness, scaling, cracking of the skin, or a ring-shaped rash may occur. If the infection involves the scalp or beard, hair may fall out. Infected nails become discolored, thick, and may possibly crumble. More serious infections may lead to an abscess or cellulitis.	Characteristic appearance, smear and culture of specimen	Azoles (for surface treatment). Griseofulvin, azoles and allylamines (for internal treatment)

Cont...

Cont...

Disease	Pathogenic Organisms	Pathogenesis	Symptoms	Diagnostic tests	Treatment
Pityriasis versicolor (a lipophilic yeast)	*Malassezia furfur*	Yeasts proliferate in settings of lipids and sweat. Rare in kids, appears in adolescence.	Patches that may be white, pink, red, or brown and can be lighter or darker than the skin around them. Spots that do not tan the way the rest of your skin does. Spots that may occur anywhere on your body but are most commonly seen on your neck, chest, back, and arms.	Characteristic appearance; UV light flourescence	Selenium sulfide or azoles
SUBCUTANEOUS FUNGAL INFECTIONS					
Sporotrichosis	*Sporothrix schenckii*	Thorny plants (roses) or splinters inoculate fungus into subcutaneous tissues. Infection spreads slowly along draining lymphatics. Tissue reaction mixed pyogenic and granulomatous.	Once the mold spores move into the skin, the disease takes days-to-months to develop. The first symptom is a firm bump (nodule) on the skin that can range in color from pink to nearly purple.	Culture of tissue or drainage (fungi rarely seen on smear or section). Skin test determines exposure but not disease.	Ketoconazole, itraconazole, Amphotericin B

Cont...

Disease	Pathogenic Organisms	Pathogenesis	Symptoms	Diagnostic tests	Treatment
PATHOGENIC FUNGAL INFECTIONS					
Histoplasmosis	*Histoplasma capsulatum*	Spores inhaled from soil, transform to yeast in lungs, phagocytosed by macrophages. May resolve, resolve with scarring, remain active in lungs, or, especially in settings of immunocompromise, disseminate. Moves throughreticuloendothelial organs (liver, spleen, lymph nodes)	Symptoms are similar to those of pneumonia and include: fever, chest pains and a dry or non- productive cough. Some people may also experience joint pain. If the disease is not treated, it can disseminate (spread) from the lungs to other organs.	Skin test confirms exposure, but not infection. Antibody titers are often unreliable, especially in immunocompromise. Organisms seen intracellularly in blood/ bone marrow/ liver/urine/ tissue and/or grown in culture.	Amphotericin B
Coccidioidomycosis (Valley Fever)	*Coccidioides immitis*	Inhaled spores swell into spherules in lung, burst releasing hundreds of endospores. Hematogenous dissemination of endospores to meninges, skin, bone, liver, spleen with lesions ranging from pyogenic abscesses to granulomas.	Symptoms of valley fever include: Fatigue (tiredness), Cough, Fever, Short- ness of breath, Headache, Night sweats, Muscle aches or joint pain, Rash on upper body or legs. In extremely rare cases, the fungal spores can enter the skin through a cut, wound, or splinter and cause a skin infection.	Coccidioidin skin test positive 1-3 weeks after infection but not reliable: anergy common in disseminated disease. Complement fixation antibody may be + in disseminated disease, but not helpful in immunocompromised hosts. Best: smear and culture of pus, tissue.	Amphotericin B; fluconazole; itraconazole.

Cont...

Cont...

Disease	Pathogenic Organisms	Pathogenesis	Symptoms	Diagnostic tests	Treatment
Blastomycosis	*Blastomyces dermatitidis*	Conidia inhaled, convert to yeast form in lungs. Dissemination via infected macrophages to skin, bone, urinary tract.	Similar to flu symptoms and include fever, chills, cough, muscle aches, joint pain, and chest pain. In very serious cases of blastomycosis, the fungus can disseminate (spread) to other parts of the body, such as the skin and bones.	No adequate skin test; antibody or antigen assays exist. Best option is smear or culture of affected site.	Amphotericin B, Ketoconazole, Itraconazole
OPPROTUNISTIC FUNGAL INFECTIONS					
Cryptococcosis	*Cryptococcus neoformans*	Aerosolized yeasts inhaled. Hematogenous dissemination to central nervous system.	Pulmonary disease (nodular, miliary) may occur. Mucoid, cloudy meninges in Central nervous system Intracerebral masses of yeasts may form (cryptococcomas).	India ink preparation, culture of cerebrospinal fluid (or other body site). Polysaccharide capsule alalows for easy cryptococcal antigen assay in serum or cerebrospinal fluid – sensitive and specific when titers are high.	Amphotericin B + 5-flucytosine Fluconazole

Cont...

Cont...

Disease	Pathogenic Organisms	Pathogenesis	Symptoms	Diagnostic tests	Treatment
Candidiasis	*Candida albicans*	Dissemination occurs via defect in mucosa, or formation of biofilm on catheter, other foreign body.	Vaginitis, dysuria, fever, chills, renal dysfunction, endophthalmitis, skin lesions.	1. Pathognomonic appearance (thrush) 2. Smear/culture of usually sterile site 3. Pathologic confirmation: organism in tissue	Nystatin, Clotrimazole, Amphotericin B, Fluconazole, Voriconazole, Caspofungin
Aspergillosis	*Aspergillus fumigatus, A. flavus*	Airborne spores are inhaled.	Symptoms of allergic bronchopulmonary aspergillosis (ABPA) may include: Wheezing, Coughing, Fever (in rare cases) Symptoms of invasive aspergillosis may include: Fever, Chest pain, Coughing, Shortness of breath, Aspergilloma, or "fungus ball"	Stain and culture of tissue biopsy specimen. (Positive culture of a secretion may represent contamination)	Corticosteroids, Amphotericin B, Itraconazole, Voriconazole, Caspofungin

Cont...

■ COMMON DISEASES CAUSED BY PROTOZOA (FIG. 9.4 AND TABLE 9.4)

Protozoa are one of the three main classes of parasites that cause diseases in humans. They are single-celled organisms and can only be seen under microscope. When they invade a human they are able to multiply easily which causes them to be at a great advantage and put humans at a disadvantage. This helps them to be survive in the human body and causes serious infection even with the arrival of a single protozoon.

Infections caused by protozoa are contagious. Those protozoa that have inhabited the human intestine can be transmitted from one human to the other via the faecal-oral route, such as through sharing food the infected person has touched and through direct person to person contact. Protozoa living in the blood or tissue can be transmitted through a third source such as mosquito. Infections are easily transmitted and persons carrying this parasite should avoid interactions with others, especially those with compromised and weakened immune systems.

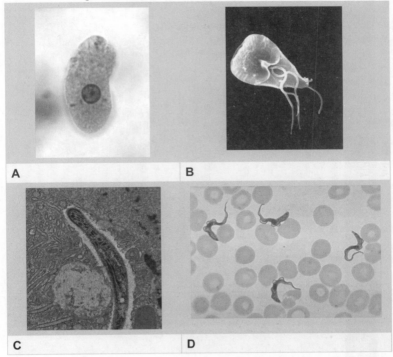

Figures 9.4 (A to D): Common protozoan parasites of human beings. (A) *Entamoeba histolytica*, causal organism of amoebiasis, (B) *Giardia lamblia*, causal organism of giardiasis, (C) *Plasmodium vivax*, causal organism of malaria, (D) *Trypanosoma brucei*, causal organism of African sleeping sickness. *(For color version see plate 8)*

Table 9.4: Common protozoan diseases

Disease	Pathogenic Agent	Transmission	Symptoms	Diagnosis	Treatment
Amoebiasis	*Entamoeba histolytica*	Usually in faeces, via water and contaminated salad and fruits	Dysentery, flatulence, loss of water, thirst, depression, gut ulceration, enlarged liver, if severe death can also occur within 4-weeks	Faeces is microscopically examined, histology of gut content is studied	Metronidazol, Diiodohydroxyquin
Giardiasis	*Giardia lamblia*	Direct infection	Bloody diarrhea, vomiting	Faeces examined	Metronidazol, Carnidazol
Malaria	*Plasmodium-*species	It spreads when an infected Anopheles mosquito bites a person. This is the only type of mosquito that can spread malaria. The mosquito becomes infected by biting an infected person and drawing blood that contains the parasite. When that mosquito bites another person, that person becomes infected.	Fever, Chills, Headache, Sweats, Fatigue, Nausea and vomiting, Back pain, Dry cough etc.	Blood test is conducted for the presence of parasite	Common antimalarial drugs include: Chloroquine, Quinine sulfate, Hydroxychloroquine

Cont...

Cont...

Disease	Pathogenic Agent	Transmission	Symptoms	Diagnosis	Treatment
Trypanosomiasis (African Sleeping sickness)	Trypanosoma species	The disease is mostly transmitted through the bite of an infected tsetse fly, Mother-to-child infection, Mechanical transmission through other blood sucking insects is also possible.	Fever, headaches, joint pains and itching, changes of behaviour, confusion, sensory disturbances and poor coordination, Disturbance of the sleep cycle	Screening for potential infection- This involves using serological tests (only available for *T.b.gambiense*) and checking for clinical signs - generally swollen cervical glands.	Pentamidine, Suramin, Melarsoprol etc

Table 9.5: Common diseases caused by mycoplasma

Diseases	Causal Agent	Transmission	Symptoms	Areas affected	Treatment and Prevention
Mycoplasma Pneumonia	*Mycoplasma pneumonia*	Mycoplasma is spread through contact with droplets from the nose and throat of infected people especially when they cough and sneeze.	Persistent fever, dry cough, bronchitis, sore throat, headache, tiredness. Infection may become dangerous and cause damage to heart and central nervous system	Respiratory tract and ears	Antibiotics such as erythromycin azithromycin, tetracycline, quinolones, etc. Corticosteroids, Immunomodulatory therapy Prevention: 6-8 hours of sleep, balanced diet, washing hands before eating or after interacting with sick patients

Cont...

Diseases	Causal Agent	Transmission	Symptoms	Areas affected	Treatment and Prevention
M. haemofilis infection	Mycoplasma haemophilis	It is transmitted via blood sucking arthropod vectors including fleas, mosquitoes and ticks.	Anaemia (infection of erythrocytes), lethargy, fever and anorexia	Blood, spleen, liver, lungs, bone marrow	Antibiotics such as Doxycyclin and Enrofloxacin are used for treatment
M. genitalium infection	Mycoplasma genitalium	Transmitted between partners during unprotected sexual intercourse.	Urethritis (in men), discharge in both sexes, burning while urinating, arthritis, vaginal itching, pain during intercourse in women.	Genitals of men and women	Antibiotics such as Azythromycin, Erythromycin, Ofloxacin, Levofloxacin, Doxycyclin are used for treatment

■ COMMON DISEASES CAUSED BY CHLAMYDIA

Chlamydia is a sexually transmitted disease (STD) caused by the bacteria *Chlamydia trachomatis*. When transmitted through sexual contact, the bacteria can infect the urinary and reproductive organs. Two other types of Chlamydia species can also lead to illness:

- *Chlamydia pneumoniae*, which can be spread through coughing and sneezing.
- *Chlamydia psittaci*, which birds can pass to humans.

Symptoms

In many cases, Chlamydia causes only mild symptoms or no symptoms at all. So an infection can last for weeks or months before it is discovered.

Symptoms include:

- burning feeling during urination
- discharge from the penis or vagina
- vaginal irritation
- pain in the lower abdomen
- painful sexual intercourse in women
- pain in the testicles in men

Untreated Chlamydia in females can lead to pelvic inflammatory disease (PID), which can affect the vagina, cervix, uterus, fallopian tubes and ovaries. Sometimes, PID causes no symptoms; more often, it causes abdominal or lower back pain, painful urination, pain during intercourse, bleeding between menstrual periods, nausea, vomiting, fatigue, or fever. It can cause scarring of the fallopian tubes which can lead to serious health problems such as chronic pelvic pain, infertility. or ectopic (tubal) pregnancy.

Untreated infections in males can lead to epididymitis, an inflammation of the coiled tubes in the back of the testicles. This can result in testicular swelling, pain and even infertility.

Transmission

Chlamydia is contagious. It can be transmitted through sexual contact via semen and vaginal secretions. Chlamydia does not spread through casual contact such as shaking hands or using the same toilet as someone who is infected.

Diagnosis

Tests can be done to find out if the bacteria that cause Chlamydia is in the body. A urine test will be taken. In case of females the cervix can also be swabbed while the urethra, where urine flows from, may be swabbed in case of males. If there is a chance, the Chlamydia is in the rectum or throat, these areas may be swabbed as well.

Treatment

If detected early Chlamydia can easily be treated with antibiotics and the symptoms alleviated within 7 to 10 days. Azithromycin is an antibiotic usually prescribed in a single dose while doxycycline must be taken twice per day for about one week.

The sexual partners of anyone who has (or is thought to have) Chlamydia or any other STD should be examined and treated. Those diagnosed with an STD should inform their partners as soon as possible so that they too can be examined and treated to prevent complications and avoid spreading the infection.

Prevention

Because Chlamydia is spread through sexual contact, the best way to prevent it is to abstain from having sex. Sexual contact with more than one partner or with someone who has more than one partner increases the risk of contracting any STD.

In addition, when properly and consistently used, condoms decrease the risk of STDs, including Chlamydia.

■ Common diseases caused by Rickettsia

Rickettsial disease encompasses a group of diseases caused by the microorganism *rickettsiae*.

The organisms cause disease by damaging blood vessels in various tissues and organs. In severe cases multiple tissues and organs are affected.

Table 9.6: Common diseases caused by rickettsia

Disease	Causative rickettsia	Transmitting vector/Carrier
Rocky Mountain spotted Fever (RMSF)	*R. rickettsia*	Vector: Wood tick, dog tic and lone star tick Humans become incidental host after being bitten by infected adult tick
Rickettsialpox	*R. akari*	Vector: House Mouse is the natural host of the mouse mite transmitting rikettsialpox Distribution: Russia, South Africa, Korea
Boutonneuse fever	*R. conorii*	Vector: Various ticks including dog ticks
Louse-borne typhus	*R. prowazekii*	Vector: Lice pedicures
Brill-Zinsser disease	*R. prowazekii*	Vector: Lice Reactivation of the organism form a latent state up to decades after primary infection
Murine	*R. typhi and R felis*	Transmitted between RATS by rat flea Humans accidentally infected by the faeces of infected fleas
Tsutsugamushi disease	*O. tsutsugamushi*	Vector: Larval trombiculid mites in soil and scrub
Q fever	*C. burnetii*	Vector: Airborne droplets from infected cattle, sheep goats, rodents and cats

Table 9.7: Symptoms of rickettsial diseases

Rickettsial disease	Characteristic signs and symptoms
RMSF	• Onset gradual or abrupt, starting about 2–8 days after a tick bite • Fever, headache, confusion, aching muscles, gastrointestinal symptoms • Rash from day 2–3 consisting of small red blotches on wrist and ankles that become widespread and sometimes blister • 20% of cases do not develop rash (spotless RMSF)
Rickettsial Pox	• Irregular fluctuating fever occurs and lasts for <1 week • Headache, chills, aching muscles, runny nose, sore throat, nausea and vomiting, • Red raised spot develops at se of mete bite, later forming a dry scab (eschar) • Rash distributed on the face, neck, trunk and extremities, and is easily confused with rash of varicella (chickenpox)
Boutonneuse fever	• Fever, headache, malaise, aching muscles • Rash appears on days 35 of illness, spreading from the extremities to the trunk neck,face, palms and soles within 36 hours • Rash is spotty and blotchy and may persist for 2–3 weeks • In half the cases, a dry scab known as a tache noire (black spot) develops
Louse-borne typhus Brill-Zinsser disease	• Abrupt onset occurring 1–2 weeks after louse bite • Fever and intractable headache. • On days 4–7 of illness, rash appears and soles are usually not affected • Rash initially splotehy, developing into raised red spots • Brill-Zinsser disease is usually milder
Murine	• Similar to louse-borne typhus but tends to have a milder and shorter course • Flea-bite does not have an eschar
Tsutsugamushi disease	• Generalised swelling of the lymph nodes is common • Fever and headache • Rash occur 1–3 weeks after a mite bite and is a dry scab-like lesion • Rash usually only around the trunk and has a short duration
Q Fever	• Onset is usually abrupt with fever, intractable headache, chills, muscle pain, cough and chest pain • Usually no rash appears • Pneumonitis (lung involvement) occurs in more than half of patients

Diagnosis

This is a blood test that detects the presence of antibodies to rickettsial antigens.

Treatment

- All rickettsial diseases should be treated with antibiotic therapy.
- Doxycycline is the drug of choice. Chloramphenicol may be used as an alternative.

■ Common Diseases caused by Spirochetes

Table 9.8: Spirochetes and the human diseases they produce

Organism	Disease
Borrelia burgdoiferi	Lyme disease
Borrelia species	Relapsing fever
	Louse-borne
	Tick-borne
Treponema pallidun pallidum	Syphilis
Treponema pallidun pertenue	Yaws
Treponema pallidun endemicum	Bejel (endemic syphilis)
Treponema carateum	Pinta
Leptospirosis interrogans	Leptospira
	Anicteric
	Icteric

■ Possible Questions

1. Give a detail account of the diseases caused by bacteria.
2. Write an essay on common diseases caused by microorganisms.
3. What is AIDS? Give an account of its causal agent, symptoms, diagnosis, treatment and prevention.
4. Give a brief note on protozoa and discuss the diseases caused by them.
5. Discuss diseases caused by chlamydia in detail.
6. Write Short Notes:
   - Mycoplasma and diseases caused
   - Diseases caused by Ricketsia
   - RMSF
   - Protozoan Parasites

Chapter

10

Infection and Transmission of Pathogenic Microorganisms

■ INTRODUCTION

An infection is caused by invasion of foreign cells like bacteria in human that causes harm to the host organism. Generally the host organism is considered "colonized" by cells that don't belong to it. These foreign cells must be harmful to the host organism the colonization be considered as an infection.

■ WHAT IS INFECTION?

Infection is invasion of a host organism's body tissues by disease-causing organisms, their multiplication, the reaction of host tissues to these organisms and the toxins they produce.

Infectious diseases are also known as transmissible or communicable diseases comprising of clinically evident illness resulted from infection.

■ SOME IMPORTANT TERMS RELATED TO INFECTION

- **Symptoms:** The subjective sign observed during a disease are called as its symptoms. Here subjective sign mean they can only be felt by the patient. For example, anxiety, back pain and fatigue (tiredness) are all symptoms which can be felt only by the patient.
- **Medical Sign:** The objective sign observed during a disease are called as its medical sign. Here objective sign mean they can be observed by the patient, physicians and others. For example, such as blood in the stool, a skin rash, etc. can be seen by all.
- **Syndrome:** This is a group of symptoms which consistently occur together. For example in Acquired Immune Deficiency Syndrome (AIDS) disease a collection of symptoms is observed in the patient.
- **Acute illness** are those that will eventually resolve without any medical supervision., e.g. Common cold.

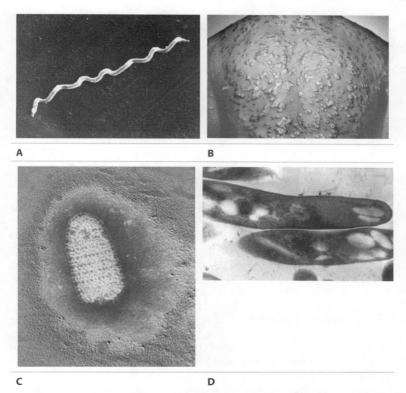

Figures 10.1 (A to D): (A) *Treponema pallidum*, the causal organism of syphilis (B) Symptoms of Syphilis (C) Rabies virus, the causal organism of rabies (D) *Mycobacterium tuberculosis*, causal organisms of tuberculosis.

- **Chronic illness** are more serious illness that require medical supervision, e.g. Tuberculosis or Cancer.

■ SOURCES OF INFECTION

The sources of infection can be divided into two main groups viz.

(a) Endogenous Sources: A Source of infection is endogenous when the infectious agent comes from the patient's own body usually from his own normal flora. Endogenous Source of infection becomes important when person's own immunity against his normal flora becomes compromised such as in case of contamination during surgery, malnutrition, impairment of blood supply and debilitating diseases such as AIDS, Diabetes or any other accompanying infection. Examples are genera of *Staphylococci* and *Streptococci* which are normally found in the body but can become pathogenic in certain circumstances.

(b) Exogenous Sources: Exogenous sources of infection introduce organisms anywhere from outside to inside of the body. In addition to being exogenous most of the time, infections are transmitted from person to person or from animal to man. To be more specific, exogenous source of infections can either be human, animal or environmental in origin.

- **Human Origin:** Human can be source of infection in three cases, (1) either when they are clinically infected (symptomatic infection), (2) when they are asymptomatically infected or (3) when they are carriers. Humen can be a source of organisms which cause diseases that are sexually transmitted such as *Treponema pallidum* that causes Syphilis and *N. gonorrhoea* that causes Gonorrheal infections. Infection may also occur through blood when vectors act as vehicles as in the case of transmission. For example, *Borrelia* that causes relapsing fever.

- **Animal Origin:** Animals are another source of infection and an infection derived from this source is called zoonotic infection. Such infections are usually maintained in animals and are acquired accidentally. An example of such infections could be Brucellosis caused by Brucella mainly from cows and their products such as milk; Rabies caused by Rabies Virus from wild animals and Plague which is caused by *Pasteurella pestis*. Moreover, animal products such as meat, milk and eggs can be sources of infection. Example: *Salmonella* species and *Campylobacter*.

- **Environmental Origin:** Environmental sources are numerous and few environmental saprophytes are pathogenic for man unless in cases of individuals with severely compromised immune system. But still some parasites may result in complications if introduced into the body from environment. Examples are *Bacillus* and *Clostridium*. Food is another important and very common source of infection due to everyday pattern of dealing with such material. Food can be contaminated and hence a source of infection at several stages. At its origin (infected animal or plant), or at the time of processing when handled with hands or contaminated tools. It is not only a vehicle when transmission is considered but it is also a good environment where bacteria or any other pathogen can multiply and produce toxins.

There is another type of infection called as nosocomial infection or hospital acquired infections. Nosocomial infection is acquired in hospitals and other healthcare facility centres. These infections can be seen in patients acquired during their stay in a healthcare facility or it can manifest after discharge. Such infections are considered more difficult to prevent and treat more unpredictable and more resistant to cure than infections contracted in the community. Patients who undergo surgical procedures have a higher incidence of nosocomial infections than others. The source of microorganisms that cause nosocomial infections can be the patients themselves, healthcare facility or the healthcare personnel.

■ CHAIN OF INFECTION

1. **In order for infection to occur in an individual, a process involving six related components must occur. This process has been referred to as the "Chain of Infection." The six steps or "links" in the chain are:**

   1. Infectious Agents
   2. Reservoir
   3. Portal of Exit
   4. Mode of Transmission
   5. Portal of Entry
   6. Susceptible Host

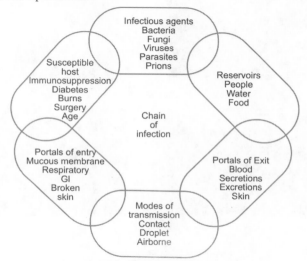

Figure 10.2: Chain of infection

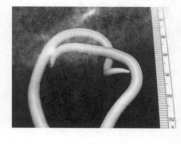
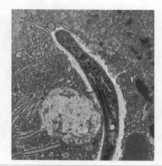

A   B

Figure 10.3 (A to I): (A) *Ascaris lumbricoides* (metazoa), causal organisms of Ascariasis, (B) *Plasmodium vivax* (Protozoa), causal organisms of Malaria, (C) *Candida albicans* (Fungi), causal organism of Candidiasis, (D) Candidiaisis, (E) *Vibrio cholerae* (Bacteria), causal organism of cholera, (F) *Rickettsia rickettsii* (Rickettsia), causal organism of rocky mountain soptted fever, (G) Rocky mountain spotted fever, (H) Human Immuno Deficiency virus (HIV), causal organisms of Acquired Immuno Deficiency syndrome (AIDS), (I) Prions, Causal agent of Kuru, BSE and CJD

■ INFECTIOUS AGENTS

There are seven categories of biological agents that can cause infectious diseases. Each has its own particular characteristics. The types of agents are:

(a) Metazoa: These are multicellular animals, most of which are parasites. They cause diseases viz:

- Trichinellosis, also called trichinosis is caused by an intestinal roundworm transmitted through undercooked meat.
- Chronic Anemia is caused by hookworms which are transmitted through faeces-contaminated water and soil. Infection results in retarded mental and physical development of children.
- Schistosomiasis is caused by a blood fluke and transmitted through contaminated water. Symptoms are related to the number and location of eggs in human body and may involve liver, intestines, spleen, urinary tract, and reproductive system.

(b) Protozoa: These are single-cell organisms with a well-defined nucleus. Some of these are human parasites. Examples of diseases caused by protozoa include:

- Malaria which is a mosquito-borne disease (that is one of the top three infectious diseases in the world) along with Tuberculosis and HIV.
- Giardiasis is an infection of the upper small intestine that causes a diarrheal illness. Outbreaks can be difficult to control especially in child care settings
- Toxoplasmosis is transmitted to humen from cats and undercooked meat. When this systemic disease infects a pregnant woman, it can cause the death of the foetus
- *Pneumocystis carinii* causes Pneumonia or PCP which is often foetal, especially in people with compromised immune systems such as those infected with HIV.

(c) Fungi: These are nonmotile, filamentous organisms that cause diseases which are very difficult to be treated. Some examples important to public health are:

- Histoplasmosis is transmitted by inhaling dust from soil that contains bird droppings. The severity varies widely with the lungs, the most common site of infection.
- Candidiasis is transmitted by contact with human patients and carriers. This fungus causes lesions on the skin or mucous membranes including "thrush" and vulvovaginitis. Symptoms can be severe in immunocompromised people.

(d) Bacteria: These are single-celled organisms that lack true nuclei. They are responsible for wide range of human diseases including:

- Tuberculosis is a chronic lung disease that is a major cause of disability and death in many parts of the world.

- Staphylococcal disease can affect almost every organ system. Severity ranges from a single pustule of impetigo through pneumonia, arthritis, endocarditis, etc. to sepsis and death.
- Chlamydia and Gonorrhea are the most widespread sexually transmitted diseases.
- Tetanus and Diphtheria are two diseases those were once major public health problems but are now well controlled through immunization.

(e) Rickettsia is a genus of bacteria usually found in the cells of lice, ticks, fleas and mites. They are smaller than most bacteria and share some characteristics of viruses. Diseases cause by rickettsia include:

- Rocky Mountain Spotted Fever, a tick-borne systemic disease that can be hard to diagnose and that leads to death in 3-5% of US cases.
- Typhus, a louse-borne rash illness with a high case-fatality rate that has occurred historically in poor living conditions brought on by war and famine.

(f) Viruses are very small, consisting of RNA or DNA core and an outer coat of protein. They can reproduce and grow only inside living cells. Many viral illness is significant to public health including:

- Influenza, a respiratory illness that contributes to development of pneumonia and occurs in annual epidemics during the winter months
- HIV (Human Immuno Deficiency Virus), that causes Acquired Immuno Deficiency Syndrome (AIDS). This severe, life-threatening pandemic disease has spreaded worldwide within the past 20–30 years.
- Rabies is spreaded to human from animal bites or scratches. Rabies is almost always fatal in human but is preventable by a vaccine.
- Measles, Mumps, Rubella, and Poliomyelitis are other diseases caused by viruses. These diseases are well controlled in the US through immunization.

(g) Prions are infectious agents that do not have any genes. They seem to consist of a protein with an aberrant structure which somehow replicates in animal or human tissues. Prions cause severe damage to the brain. Diseases associated with prions include:

- Chronic Wasting Disease (CWD) seen in Mule, Deer and Elk
- Bovine Spongiform Encephalopathy (BSE) seen in Cows
- Creutzfeld-Jacob Disease (CJD) seen in human

■ RESERVOIRS

Next essential link in the chain of infection is reservoir, usual habitat in which the agent lives and multiplies. Depending upon the agent, the reservoirs may be:

(a) Human Reservoirs

There are two types of human reservoirs

1. **Acute clinical cases:** Acute clinical cases are people who are infected with the disease agent and become ill.
- **Carriers:** They are people who carry infectious agents but are not ill. Depending on the disease, any of the following types of carriers may be of following types;
  - **Incubatory carriers** are people who are going to become ill, but begin transmitting their infection before their symptoms start. Examples, Measles: a person infected with Measles begins to shed the Virus in nasal and throat secretions a day or two before any cold symptoms or rash are noticeable.
  - **Inapparent carriers:** People with inapparent infections never develop an illness, but are able to transmit their infection to others. Example, Of every 100 individuals infected with the Poliomyelitis virus, only one becomes paralyzed. Four others will have a mild illness with fever, malaise, headache, nausea and vomiting. But 95 out of the 100 will have no symptoms at all although they pass the virus in their faeces.
  - **Convalescent carriers** are people who continue to be infectious during and even after their recovery from illness. Example, Salmonella patients may excrete the bacteria in faeces for several weeks and rarely even for a year or more. This is the most common in infants and young children.
  - **Chronic carriers** are people who continue to harbour infections for a year or longer after their recovery. Example, the Chronic carrier state is not uncommon following Hepatitis B infection, whether or not the person became ill and may be lifelong.

(b) Animal Reservoirs

Animal reservoirs of infectious agents can be described in the same way as human reservoirs. They may be
- Acute clinical cases or
- Carriers

Depending upon the disease different carrier phases may be important in transmission.

(c) Environmental Reservoirs

Plants, soil and water may serve as reservoir of infection for a variety of diseases.
Examples:
- The organism that causes Histoplasmosis lives in soil with high organic content and undisturbed bird droppings.
- The agents that cause Tetanus, Anthrax and Botulism are widely distributed in soil.
- The agent of Legionnaire's disease lives in water including hot water heaters.

■ PORTAL OF EXIT

Next link in the chain of disease transmission is Portal of exit. Portal of exit is the route by which the disease agent may escape from human or animal reservoir. While many disease agents have only one portal of exit, others may leave by various portals.

The portals most commonly associated with human and animal diseases are:

(a) Respiratory: This is the route of many disease agents that cause respiratory illnesses such as the Common Cold, Influenza, and Tuberculosis. It is also the route used by many childhood Vaccine-preventable diseases, including Measles, Mumps, Rubella, Pertussis, *Haemophilus influenzae* type b (Hib) and Pneumococcal disease. This is the most important portal and the most difficult to control.

(b) Genitourinary: This portal of exit is the route of sexually transmitted diseases including Syphilis, Gonorrhoea, Chlamydia, and HIV. Schistosomiasis-a parasitic disease and Leptospirosis- a bacterial infection, are both spread through urine released into the environment.

(c) Alimentary: The alimentary portal of exit may be the mouth, as in rabies and other diseases transmitted by bites. More commonly, disease agents are spread by the other end of intestinal tract. These are referred to as enteric diseases. In general, enteric diseases may be controlled through good hygiene, proper food preparation and sanitary sewage disposal. Examples include:

- Hepatitis A
- Typhoid
- Cholera
- Giardiasis

(d) Skin: Skin may serve as a portal of exit through superficial lesions or through percutaneous penetration.

- Superficial skin lesions that produce infectious discharges are found in Smallpox, Varicella (chickenpox), Syphilis, Chancroid, and Impetigo.
- Percutaneous exit occurs through mosquito bites (Malaria, West Nile virus) or through the use of needles (Hepatitis B and C, HIV).

(e) Transplacental: This portal of exit from mother to fetus is important in the transmission of microorganisms such as Rubella, HIV, Syphilis and Cytomegalovirus (the most common infectious cause of developmental disabilities). It is fortunately not a factor for most diseases.

■ MODE OF TRANSMISSION

A mode of transmission is necessary to bridge the gap between the portal of exit from the reservoir and portal of entry into the host. Two basic modes are direct and indirect.

(a) Direct transmission: Occurs more or less immediately. Many diseases are transmitted by direct contact with the human, animal or environmental reservoir. Prime examples are sexually transmitted diseases and enteric diseases caused by *Shigella* and *Campylobacter*. Contact with soil may lead to mycotic (fungal) diseases. Droplet spread is also considered direct transmission. Infectious aerosols produced by coughing or sneezing can transmit infection directly to susceptible people up to three feet away. Many respiratory diseases are spread this way.

(b) Indirect transmission: May occur through animate or inanimate mechanisms.

- **Animate mechanisms:** Involve vectors. Flies may transmit infectious agents such as *Shigella* in a purely mechanical way by walking on faeces and then on food. Mosquitoes, ticks or fleas may serve as reservoirs for the growth and multiplication of agents, for example in Malaria or Lyme disease.
- **Inanimate mechanisms:** When disease agents are spread by environmental vehicles or by air, this is referred to as indirect transmission by inanimate mechanisms. Anything may be a vehicle, including objects, food, water, milk, or biological products.
  - Food is a common vehicle for Salmonella infections
  - Water is the usual vehicle in Cholera outbreaks
  - Surgical instruments and implanted medical devices may be the vehicles of *Staphylococcal* infections

■ PORTALS OF ENTRY

The point where infectious agent enters new host is known as the portal of entry such as:

- Non-intact skin, e.g. broken skin such as bed sores or wounds coming in contact with contaminated material
- Respiratory tract, e.g. inhaling air having pathogen
- Gastrointestinal tract, e.g. eating contaminated food
- Mucous membranes, e.g. eyes, nose or mouth exposures with infectious agents

■ SUSCEPTIBLE HOST

All individuals may be susceptible depending on the exposure and their own general health status. Individuals who have never been exposed to the Organism may become ill because they do not have antibodies to protect them (e.g. communicable diseases) either through immunization or previous infection.

Factors that increase the risk of susceptibility are:

- Age (either very young or very old)
- Underlying medical conditions
- Treatments or invasive devices
- Poor nutrition/general health

■ POSSIBLE QUESTIONS

1. What are the different modes of entry of microorganisms into the body?
2. Define infection and classify it.
3. Write an essay on transmission of infection.
4. What are different types of sources of infection?
5. Explain about the mode of transmission of infection.
6. What are the principles of infection control?
7. **Write Short Notes:**
   - Susceptible host
   - Portals of entry
   - Direct and Indirect modes of disease transmission
   - Portals of exit
   - Carriers
   - Infectious agent
   - Chain of infection
   - Endogenous and exogenous sources of infection
   - Syndrome and symptom
   - Acute and chronic illness
   - Reservoir

Chapter

11

Collection of Specimen by Nurses

■ INTRODUCTION

One means of gathering information about patient's health status is by identifying pathogens and analyzing urine, blood, sputum, and faeces. Nurses are responsible for collecting and labeling specimen for analysis and ensuring their delivery to the laboratory.

■ WHAT IS A SPECIMEN?

A specimen is a sample collected from patient's tissue, fluid or other material for laboratory analysis. This is necessary to carry out medical diagnosis of a disease.

Common examples of specimen include:

- Throat swabs
- Sputum
- Urine
- Blood
- Surgical drain fluids
- Tissue biopsies

■ PRINCIPLES OF SPECIMEN COLLECTION

A laboratory depends on nurses to collect specimen in an accurate manner. The welfare of patient rests not only on laboratory analysis and physician's interpretation but also on the way in which a specimen is obtained and transmitted to the laboratory by nurses. Factors that must be considered while collecting specimens are as follows;

(a) Moisture: Moist specimens must always be submitted to a laboratory for analysis. Most bacteria cannot survive in a dry environment, especially the pathogenic ones. Dry swabs are of no value. Hence, when a specimen is taken a nurse must be sure the swab is moist and then delivered to laboratory immediately before it dries out.

(b) Time of Collection: Specimens must be taken possibly before antibiotics are administered. If antibiotics have already been started, then the laboratory sheet must be marked so that everyone is aware of. The timing of blood specimen is very important. Detection of positive blood culture depends on the pathogenic process of the organism.

(c) Labeling and Handling of Containers: All containers used for specimen collection must be sterile. The patient should be instructed to handle the container as aseptically as possible, i.e. not to touch the inside of container, laying the lid down in such a way as to contaminate it, leaving the lid off for an excessive length of time, etc. If any of the specimen is spilled on outside, it should immediately be cleaned with a disinfectant. The lid should be secured tightly and the container transported with care to insure against spillage. All containers must be labeled clearly with the patient's name, hospital number, room number and the source of specimen. All specimens are to be sent in ziplock bags to the laboratory. It is absolutely necessary that the specimen be accompanied by a requisition sheet completely filled out which should include information on the specimen container as well as physician, examinations requested, time specimen was collected, clinical diagnosis, current antibiotic therapy. Specimens and sheets improperly identified should be refused by the laboratory.

(d) Effect of Temperature: Most of the microorganisms found in clinical specimens have an optimal temperature of 37°C. Most have a broad range of temperature tolerance; however, some very important pathogens die rapidly when subjected to temperature below their optimal requirement. Therefore, it is better never to refrigerate any specimen especially spinal fluids, vaginal and urethral discharges but deliver them immediately to the laboratory after collection.

(e) Effect of atmosphere: The atmosphere plays a very important role in isolating and identifying pathogenic bacteria. The two principal gases that affect metabolism of the bacteria are Oxygen and Carbon dioxide. Some bacteria require Oxygen, some require small amounts with varying concentration of Carbon dioxide and some, the anaerobes, must have an atmosphere completely devoid of any trace of Oxygen. Again, it is most important to get the specimen to the laboratory immediately. Anaerobic Organisms must be placed in an Oxygen-free environment within 30 minutes after collection.

General Considerations For Specimen Collection

- Collect specimen before antibiotic therapy whenever possible.
- Collect material from where the suspected organism will most likely be found.

- Observe asepsis in collection of all specimens.
- Consider the stage of disease.
- Instruct patients clearly.
- Use proper containers and/or transport media.
- Deliver specimen promptly.
- Provide sufficient information to the laboratory.

■ THROAT CULTURE (FIGURE 11.1)

A sample of mucous and secretions from back of the throat is collected on a cotton-tipped applicator and applied to a slide or culture. A determination of which drug is most effective against a particular organism may also be done. A full culture and sensitivity test takes several days because the organisms must have time to grow.

When to Perform?

A throat culture or Strep test is performed by using a throat swab to detect the presence of group of *Streptococcus* bacteria, the most common cause of strep throat. These bacteria can also cause other infections, including pneumonia, tonsillitis, and meningitis.

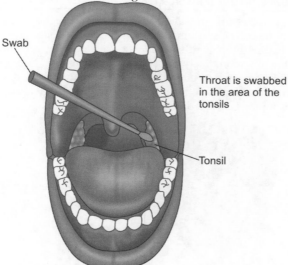

Figure 11.1: Taking sample for throat culture

Supplies and Equipment

The supplies and equipments required to obtain a sample for throat culture are:

- Sterile cotton-tipped applicator specimen collection kit.

- Tongue depressor.
- Laboratory request form.
- Flashlight.

Procedure for a Throat Culture

Always wash your hands before the procedure. Explain to the patient what you are going to do. Have the patient sit comfortably on a bed or chair and tilt his head back.

- Use flashlight to illuminate the back of the throat. Check for inflamed areas using tongue depressor.
- Ask the patient to say "Ahhh" as you swab the tonsil areas from side to side. Be sure to include any inflamed sites.
- Avoid touching the tongue, cheeks or teeth with the applicator as this will contaminate it with oral bacteria.
- Place the cotton-tipped applicator into the culture tube immediately.
- Label culture tube with the patient's name, SSN, and ward number if applicable.
- Complete the request form.

■ SPUTUM CULTURE (FIGURE 11.2)

Sputum is a mixture of saliva and mucous coughed up from the respiratory tract. The sputum specimen should be collected early in the morning before the patient eats, brushes his teeth or uses mouthwash. The specimen is more likely to contain sputum at this time rather than just saliva. Specimens are often taken for three consecutive days because it is difficult for the patient to cough up enough sputum at one time and an organism may be missed if only one culture is done.

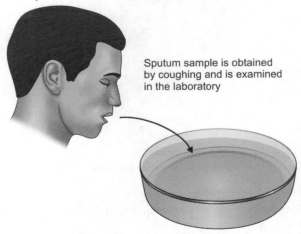

Sputum sample is obtained by coughing and is examined in the laboratory

Figure 11.2: Taking sample for sputum culture

When to perform?

A sputum culture is done to:
- find and identify bacteria or fungi that are causing an infection (such as Pneumonia or Tuberculosis) of the lungs.
- identify the best antibiotic to treat the infection (sensitivity testing).
- monitor treatment of an infection.

Supplies and Equipments

Supplies and equipments required to collect a sputum specimen are
- Sterile container with tight-fitting lid.
- Box of tissues.
- Gloves.
- Laboratory request form.

Procedure for Sputum Specimen

- Wash your hands and gather the equipment.
- Explain the procedure to the patient.
- Place the tissues nearby and have the patient rinse his mouth with clear water to remove any food particles.
- Assist the patient to a sitting position. If necessary ask him to cough deeply and spit into the container. Tell the patient to avoid touching inside of the container because it is sterile.
- A sputum specimen is considered to be highly contaminated and must be treated with caution. To prevent contamination by particles in air, keep the container closed until the patient is ready to spit into it. Close the container immediately after collecting the specimen to prevent the spread of any organisms from the Specimen. Offer tissues for the patient to wipe his mouth.
- Wash your hands, label the container and complete the laboratory request form. Take the specimen to the laboratory immediately allowing it to remain in a warm place which will result in overgrowth of any organisms that may be present.
- Record the amount, consistency and colour of the sputum collected, as well as the time and date in the nursing notes.

■ STOOL SPECIMEN

A stool analysis is a series of tests done on a stool (faeces) sample to help diagnose certain conditions affecting the digestive tract. These conditions can include infection (such as from parasites, viruses or bacteria), poor nutrient absorption, or cancer.

When to perform?

Stool analysis is done to:
- help identifying diseases of digestive tract, liver, and pancreas.

- help finding the cause of symptoms affecting digestive tract, including prolonged diarrhoea, bloody diarrhoea, an increased amount of gas, nausea, vomiting, loss of appetite, bloating, abdominal pain and cramping and fever.
- screen for colon cancer by checking for hidden (occult) blood.
- look for parasites such as pinworms or Giardia.
- look for the cause of an infection such as bacteria, a fungus, or a virus.
- check for poor absorption of nutrients by the digestive tract (malabsorption syndrome).

Supplies and Equipments

Supplies and equipments required to collect a stool specimen are
- Gloves
- Clean bedpan and cover (an extra bedpan or urinal if the patient must void).
- Specimen container and lid.
- Wooden tongue blades.
- Paper bag for used tongue blades.
- Labels.
- Plastic bag for transport of container with specimen to the laboratory.

Procedure for Stool Specimen

- Explain the reason for the test and procedure to patient. Ask the patient to tell you when he feels the urge to have a bowel movement.
- Wear gloves when handling any bodily discharge.
- Give the bedpan when the patient is ready. If the patient wants to urinate first, give a male the urinal or give a female the extra bedpan.
- Remove the bedpan. Use the tongue blade to transfer a portion of the faeces to the specimen container. Do not touch the specimen because it is contaminated. It is not necessary to keep this specimen sterile however because the gastrointestinal tract is not sterile.
- Cover the container and label it with the patient's name and social security number.
- Complete the appropriate laboratory request form, noting any special examination ordered.
- Take the specimen to the laboratory immediately; examination for parasites, ova and organisms must be made while the stool is warm.

■ URINE SPECIMENS

Simple urine tests, such as for sugar and acetone, are often performed by the nurse in the hospital or by the patient at home.

When to perform?

- Urine tests are very useful for providing information to assist in the diagnosis, monitoring and treatment of a wide range of diseases.

- In addition, a urine test can determine whether or not a woman is ovulating or pregnant.
- Urine can also be tested for a variety of substances relating to drug abuse, both as part of rehabilitation program and in the world of professional sport.
- The urine can be tested very quickly using a strip of special paper which is dipped in the urine just after urination.
- This will show if there are any abnormal products in the urine such as sugar, protein, or blood.
- If more tests are needed to get more details, the urine will be analyzed in a laboratory.

Physical Appearance Test

Urine is assessed first for its physical appearance:

a. Colour: Freshly voided urine is transparent and light amber in colour. The amount and kinds of waste in the urine make it lighter or darker. Blood in the urine colours it. If the amount of blood in the urine is great, the urine will be red.

b. Odour: Freshly voided urine has a characteristic odour. When urine stands, decomposition from bacterial activity gives it an ammonia-like odour. Refrigerate the urine sample if it is not to be examined at once.

Midstream Urine Specimen

Midstream urine collection is the most common method of obtaining urine specimens from adults, particularly men. This method allows a specimen which is not contaminated from external sources to be obtained without catheterization.

a. Supplies and Equipments

- Sterile specimen cup
- Zephiran, a soap solution
- Three cotton balls (to use with zephiran or soap solution)
- Laboratory request form

b. Procedure

- Instruct the patient to clean urethral area thoroughly. This will prevent external bacteria from entering the specimen. The female should wipe from front to back to avoid contaminating the vaginal and urethral area from anal area. She should clean each side with a separate cotton ball then use the last one for the urethral area itself. The male should cleanse the penis using the first cotton ball for the urethral, the next cotton ball to clean the end of the penis and the last to cleanse the urethral opening.
- Instruct the patient to void a small amount of urine into the toilet to rinse out the urethra, void the midstream urine into the specimen

cup and the last of the stream into the toilet. The midstream urine is considered to be bladder and kidney washings; the portion that the physician wants to be tested.

- Complete the laboratory request form, label the specimen container with patient identifying information and send to the laboratory immediately. A delay in examining the specimen may cause a false result when bacterial determinations are to be made.
- Wash your hands and instruct the patient to do likewise.
- Record that the specimen was collected. Note any difficulties the patient had or if the urine had an abnormal appearance.

24-hours Urine Specimen

A 24-hours urine collection always begins with an empty bladder so that the urine collected is not "left over" from previous hours. This specimen shows the total amounts of wastes the kidneys are eliminating and the amount of each.

a. Supplies and Equipments

- Large, clean bottle with cap or stopper
- Measuring graduate
- Bedpan or urinal
- Refrigerated storage area
- Gloves

b. Procedure

- Label the bottle with patient identifying information, the date and note the time of collection at beginning and end.
- Instruct the patient to void all urine into a bedpan or urinal. Measure each specimen of urine voided and pour into the refrigerated bottle. Wash your hands before and after each collection. Record each amount on the intake and output (I & O) sheet.
- Exactly 24-hours after beginning the collection, ask the patient to void. This will complete the specimen collection.
- Send the bottle and laboratory request form to the laboratory.

■ BLOOD CULTURES (FIGURE 11.3)

Blood cultures are done to identify a disease-causing organism, especially in patients who have an elevated temperature for an unknown reason. Drawing blood from HIV positive patients is done in accordance with the hospital or clinic's local policy.

When to Perform?

Blood test is performed for:
- Knowing general state of health
- Confirming the presence of a bacterial or viral infection

- Seeing how well certain organs, such as the liver and kidneys, are functioning.
- Screening for certain genetic conditions such as cystic fibrosis or spinal muscular atrophy

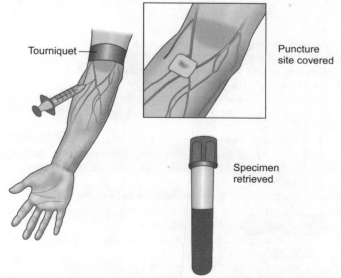

Figure 11.3: Collection of blood sample for testing

Supplies and Equipments

Supplies and equipments required for a blood culture are
- Sterile syringe (20 cc) and three needles (usually 20 gauge)
- Two blood culture bottles (one for anaerobic and one for aerobic specimens)
- Betadine solution
- Sterile cotton balls or gauze pads
- Gloves
- Tourniquet
- Band-aid
- Chux (to protect the bed)
- Laboratory request form.

Procedure for Blood Cultures

- Explain the procedure and the reason for doing such to the patient.
- Gather all supplies and equipments and bring to the patient's bedside.
- Assist the patient to a comfortable position. If the patient is noncooperative or disoriented, get someone to help you.

- Carefully wash your hands
- Clean the top of both culture bottles with betadine solution.
- Put the needle on the syringe.
- Apply the tourniquet.
- Put on gloves and clean the drawing site with betadine solution.
- Draw at least 10 cc of blood from the patient (5 cc is needed for each bottle).
- Loosen the tourniquet.
- Remove the syringe and needle while applying pressure to the venipuncture site with cotton ball or gauze pad. Have the patient apply pressure to the site.
- Replace needle on the syringe with another sterile needle.
- Inject 5 cc of blood into anaerobic bottle; do not allow air to enter the bottle.
- Replace needle on the syringe with another sterile needle.
- Inject 5 cc of blood into the aerobic bottle and while the needle is still in the bottle, disconnect it from the syringe so that air enters the aerobic bottle.
- Gently mix the blood with the solution in both bottles.
- Label both bottles with patient identifying information and the type of culture that is, (aerobic or anaerobic).
- Complete laboratory request forms and send the specimens to the laboratory immediately.
- Place a band-aid over the patient's venipuncture site.

■ POSSIBLE QUESTIONS

1. **What are Specimens? Give a detail account of the principles for collection of Specimens.**
2. **Give a detail account of the process of urine specimen collection.**
3. **What is Sputum? When we take sputum specimen for laboratory testing? Discuss its steps.**
4. **Write an essay on the procedure and precautions involved in the collection of blood sample.**
5. **Write Short Notes:**
   - Specimen collection
   - Throat culture
   - Fecal culture
   - Urine test
   - Blood test
   - Sputum culture

Chapter

12

Immunity

■ INTRODUCTION

Our body is constantly under attack by bacteria, fungi, viruses and other dangerous pathogenic organisms. But we remain healthy most of the time only because we have a good defence system within our body which is referred as the Immune system. Immunity (derived from latin term Immunis, meaning exempt) is the ability of an organism to resist infection by pathogens or state of protection against foreign organisms or substances called as antigens. Various cells, tissues and organs that carry out this activity constitute the immune system.

■ TYPES OF IMMUNITY (FLOW CHART 12.1)

Humans have two types of Immunity: Innate (Non Specific) and Adaptive (Specific). There are three line of defence systems that the organisms has to cross to invade the host (humans).
- First line of Defence (Physical and Chemical Barriers)
- Second Line of Defence (Blood and Lymph systems, cellular defences and molecular defences)
- Third Line of Defense (T-Lymphocytic cells and B-Lymphocytic cells)

■ INNATE IMMUNITY

The type of immunity inherited by the organism from parents and protects it from birth throughout life is known as Innate or Inborn Immunity. Everyone is born with innate (or natural) immunity, a type of general protection. Innate immunity acts as the first line of defence which prevents pathogens or infectious agents from entering the body.
Innate Immunity includes:

- First Line of Defence
  a. Physical barriers
  b. Chemical barriers
- Second Line of Defence
  a. Blood and Lymph systems
  b. Cellular Defences
  c. Molecular Defences

Note: Innate Immunity is also called as Non-specific or natural immunity

Flow chart 12.1: Types of immunity

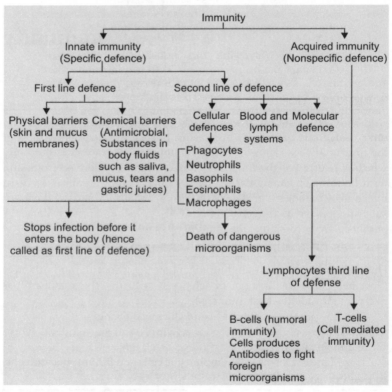

PHYSICAL BARRIERS

(a) Skin

- The Outermost layer of the skin is composed of Epithelial cells that have been keratinized meaning that they have become compacted, cemented together and filled with an insoluble protein called keratin.

Keratin doesn't normally allow the penetration of bacteria and viruses through it.

- Continuous shedding (desquamation) of the outer squamous Epithelial cells within the skin removes organisms that try to enter the skin
- Relative dryness on the skin also slows microbial growth
- Secretions from Sebaceous and Sweat glands keep the skin acidic in a pH range of 3 to 5. This acidic pH kills most microbes
- Normal flora present on skin exert their inhibitory effects on harmful pathogens

(b) Mucous Membranes

- Mucus membranes are like digestive, respiratory, and genitourinary tracts
- Prevents entry of harmful microbes
- Mucous (a viscous fluid) traps microbes and particles
- In the trachea, ciliated epithelial cells sweep out mucous, trap microbes and prevents these from entering the lungs
- Exposes them to the acidic environment of the stomach that kills most microbes

■ CHEMICAL BARRIERS

- Microbial colonization is also inhibited by Saliva, tears, and mucus secretions that continually released on exposed epithelium. All of these secretions contain antimicrobial proteins. For example: lysozyme, an enzyme found in tears, digests the cell walls of many bacteria.
- Sweat has high acid and electrolyte concentrations and this acidic pH is inhibitory to many microbes.
- The HCL in the stomach renders protection against pathogens that are swallowed. The intestine's digestive juices and bile are potentially destructive to microbes too.
- Even semen contains an antimicrobial chemical (spermine) that inhibits bacteria and the vagina has a protective acidic pH maintained by the normal flora.
- Urine has a low pH and the presence of urea and other metabolic end products (Uric acid, Fatty acids, Enzymes)

■ BLOOD AND LYMPH SYSTEMS

Two interrelated fluid systems support the body's immune response - the blood system and the lymphatic system. These two systems provide a transportation network for the cellular defences against infection.

(1) Blood System

- The blood system produces body's leukocytes (White Blood Cells) and transports these immune cells to the sites of infection (Figure 12.1, Tables 12.1 and 12.2)
- These cells circulate in the blood and are moved between arteries, capillaries and veins by the pumping of heart
- Leukocytes are defensive cells that are important to both specific and nonspecific host defences. These cells are divided into two groups: polymorphonuclear leukocytes or granulocytes and mononuclear leukocytes or agranulocytes:
  - Granulocytes- Basophils, Neutrophils and Eosinophils
  - Agranulocytes – Lymphocytes (B-Cells and T-cells). These are the third line of defence system.

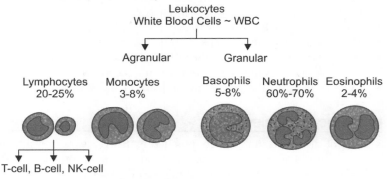

Figure 12.1: Types of leukocytes

Table 12.1: Cells of leukocytes and their functions

Leukocytes	% in WBC count	Function	Carry out Phagocytosis (engulfment of foreign proteins)
Granulocytes (have prominent cytoplasmic granules)			
Neutrophils	Makes upto 55-90%	These cells carry digestive enzymes and chemicals for phagocytosis	Yes.
Eosinophils	1-3%	High level of these cells is seen in parasitic and fungal infections. Contain digestive enzymes to kill foreign particles.	Yes, weakly phagocytic.

Cont...

Cont...

Leukocytes	% in WBC count	Function	Carry out Phagocytosis (engulfment of foreign proteins)
Basophils	Comprise of < 0.5%	Associated with allergy and inflammation reactions	No
Mast Cells		Not found in circulation and are located in tissues near blood vessels and nerves. They release chemicals such as Histamine and Serotonin	No.
Agranulocytes (Consists of Lymphocytes and Natural Killer cells- The Third line of Defence, that comes under Adaptive or Specific Immunity)			
B-cells	Lymphocytes Comprises of 20-30% of WBCs	Producers of antibodies	No. It provides specific Immunity
T-cells		Recognize foreign particles (antigens)	No. It provides specific Immunity
Natural Killer cells	5-10% of lymphoid cells	Recognize and kill infected cells	Yes
Monocytes (when mature and capable of phagocytosis, these cells are called as macrophages)	Largest of all WBC and the third most common in circulation (3-7%)	Cleaning up messes caused by infections and inflammation-even self tissues that are injured. Contains various enzymes and reactive oxygen species to kill engulfed microorganisms	Yes. Very effectively performs phagocytosis

(2) Lymphatic System

- The lymph system is a secondary transport system that serves to protect and maintain the internal fluid environment by producing and filtering lymph
- Lymph is a clear fluid that contains White Blood Cells and arises from the drainage of fluid from the bloodstream and surrounding tissue
- The fluid is filtered at points called lymph nodes - where pathogens are removed before returning to venous circulation
- Major lymphatic organs include the spleen, thymus, tonsils and adenoids.

Table 12.2: Primary functions of important immune cells

	Basophils and mast cells	Neutrophils	Eosinophils	Monocytes and macrophages	Lymphocytes and plasma cells	Dendritic cells
Primary function(s)	Release chemicals that mediate inflammation	Ingest and destroy invaders	Destroy invaders, particularly antibody-coated parasites	Ingest and destroy invaders antigen presentation	Specific responses to invaders, including antibody production	Recognize pathogens and activate other immune cells by antigen presentation

■ CELLULAR DEFENCES

The cellular defences of the innate immune system describe the types of cells employed along with the processes initiated by these cells. These defences include inflammation (by mast cells), phagocytosis, fever and clotting (by platelets).

(a) Inflammation (Figure 12.2)

- The inflammatory response is the way in which the body reacts when pathogens damage cells.
- When tissue damage occurs, mast cells release a chemical called histamine, which causes local vasodilation and increased capillary permeability.
- It also releases chemotactic factors which recruit wandering macrophages (phagocytes) to the site of damage to fight the infection.
- While inflammation is necessary to allow immune cells to access infected tissue, side effects include redness, swelling, heat and pain.
- Inflammation can either be short-term (acute) or long-term (chronic).

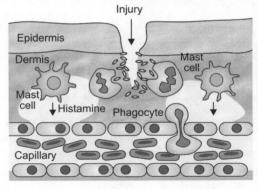

Figure 12.2: Overview of the inflammatory response. Histamine release by mast cells leading to inflammation

(b) Phagocytosis (Figure 12.3)

- Phagocytic leucocytes circulate in the blood but may move into body tissue in response to infection.
- They concentrate at sites of infection due to the release of chemicals (such as histamine) from damaged body cells.
- Pathogens are engulfed when cellular extensions (pseudopodia) surround the pathogen and then fuse, sequestering it in an internal vesicle.
- The vesicle may then fuse with the lysosome to digest the pathogen

- Some of the pathogens antigenic fragments may be presented on the surface of the macrophage, in order to help stimulate antibody production.
- This mechanism of endocytosis is called phagocytosis ('cell-eating').

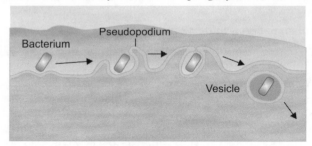

Figure 12.3: Overview of phagocytosis by a leucocyte

Phagocytic Cells

(i) Macrophages

- Large, long-lived phagocytes
- Cells extend long pseudopodia, engulf the microbe into a vacuole which fuses with a lysosome.
- Lysosomes kill in two ways
  - by generating Toxins such as Nitric oxide
  - by digetsing microbes with lysozyme
- Some microbes have outer capsules to which macrophages cannot attach. Others, like *Mycobacterium tuberculosis*, are resistant to lysosomal destruction.

(ii) Eosinophils

- Help fight large parasitic invaders, e.g. *Schistosoma mansoni* (blood fluke)
- They position themselves alongside the parasite and discharge destructive enzymes from cytoplasmic granules

(iii) Neutrophils

- Usually the first to arrive
- Attracted to chemical signals released by infected tissue
- Self-destruct while destroying invaders

(c) Fever

- A fever is an abnormally high body temperature associated with infection and is triggered by the release of prostaglandins.
- Fever may help to combat infection by reducing the growth rate of pathogens (via the inactivation of enzymes and toxins required by the invader).
- It may also increase metabolic activity of body cells and activate heat shock proteins in order to strengthen the overall immune response.
- Up to a certain point fever may be beneficial but beyond a tolerable limit it can cause damage to a body's own enzymes.

(d) Blood Clotting (Figure 12.4)

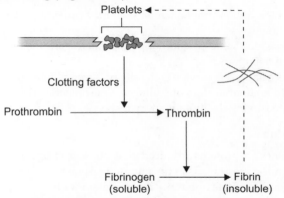

Figure 12.4: Mechanism of blood clotting

- Clotting (hemostasis) is a mechanism that prevents the loss of blood from broken vessels.
- Damaged cells and platelets release chemical signals called clotting factors which trigger a coagulation cascade.
- Clotting factors convert the inactive zymogen prothrombin into the activated enzyme thrombin.
- Thrombin catalyses the conversion of the soluble plasma protein fibrinogen into an insoluble form (fibrin).
- Fibrin forms an insoluble mesh of fibres that trap blood cells at the site of damage.
- Clotting factors also cause platelets to become sticky, which then adhere to the damaged region to form a solid plug called a clot
- The clot prevents further blood loss and blocks entry to foreign pathogens.

■ MOLECULAR DEFENCES

Molecular defences involves a number of proteins that either attack invading microbes directly or hinder their ability to reproduce.

These defences include complement proteins, cytokinetics and interferons

(a) Complement Proteins

- Complement proteins are produced by macrophages, monocytes and other body cells (particularly liver cells).
- These proteins are normally inactive in the blood but in response to immune activation initiate a cascade of reactions that help protect the body.
- Activation of the complement system may provide protection in the following ways:
    - Assist in the destruction of pathogenic organisms by destroying cell membranes.
    - Recruiting phagocytes to the site of infection (chemotaxis).
    - Aid in identification of pathogens (opsonization).
    - Intensifying the inflammatory response.

(b) Cytokines

- Cytokines are proteins produced in response to antigens and function as chemical messengers in the immune response
- They may facilitate immunity in three main ways:
    - They may regulate the innate immune response (via chemotaxis and activation of the inflammatory response)
    - They may regulate the adaptive immune response (via activation of lymphocytes)
    - They may activate hematopoiesis (production and differentiation of new white blood cells)

(c) Interferons

- Interferons are a specific type of cytokine that provide protection against viruses and tumor cells.
- Infected cells release interferons which alert surrounding cells to reduce their susceptibility to infection (e.g. by activating antiviral agents).
- Interferons will also recruit natural killer cells (NK cells) which target and destroy infected cells.

ADAPTIVE IMMUNE SYSTEM: THIRD LINE OF DEFENCE (FLOW CHARTS 12.2 AND 12.3)

The secondkind of protection is adaptive (or specific) immunity, which develops throughout our lives. This is also called as acquired immunity. Adaptive immunity involves the lymphocytes and develops as people are exposed to diseases or immunized against diseases through vaccination

Flow chart 12.2: Types of adaptive immunity

Active	Passive	Active	Passive
Antigens enter the body naturally; body induces antibodies and specialized lymphocytes	Antibodies pass from mother to fetus via placenta or to infant via the mother's milk	Antigens are introduced in vaccines; body produces antibodies and specialized lymphocytes	Preformed antibodies in immune serum are introduced by injection
(few years – life long)	(weeks - months)	(few years – life long)	(~ 3 weeks)

Natural= Normal Environmental exposure
Artificial= Medically provided

Active: Immune response, antibody production and T-cell activation
Passive: Delivery of Preformed antibodies, not long term immunity, no development of an everlasting immune response

Adaptive immune system is responsible for the destruction of foreign particles (antigens) once they have entered the body. The cells of the acquired immune system are mainly the B-cells and T-cells.

Flow chart 12.3: Classification of adaptive immunity

Humoral and Cellular Immunity

Adaptive immunity has two components: B-cells producing antibodies and T-cells both of which protect against infection. Antibodies are proteins that are produced by B-cells, circulate in the blood and bind to antigens on infectious agents. This interaction can result in direct inactivation of the microorganisms. Antibodies are primarily responsible for protection against many bacteria and viruses. This part of the immune response is termed as Humoral Immunity. B-cells produce specialized subpopulations of memory cells and plasma cells. Memory cells are capable of remembering the specific antigen and respond more rapidly and efficiently against future infections. Memory cells are long lived where as plasma cells are short lived. Plasma cells produce antibodies in the blood.

◼ ANTIBODIES (FIGURE 12.5)

Antibodies are antigen-reactive glyco-proteins, designated as immuno-globulins, present in the plasma and in extracellular fluids. They bind to specific antigens and potentially neutralize their harmful effects.

- The Ig monomer is a "Y"-shaped molecule that consists of four polypeptide chains; two identical heavy chains (H) and two identical light chains (L) connected by Disulfide bonds.

- Each heavy and light chain is made-up of a number of domains (i.e Ig folding or Ig domain).
- Each domain is about 110 Amino acids in length and contains an interchain Disulfide bond.
- Each chain in antibody consists of two regions- Constant (C) and Variable (V) region. Amino acid sequence in the C-terminal regions of the H and L chains is the same whereas the amino acid sequence in the variable region of H and L chains is different.
- The regions of variable domains actually contact the antigen and hence make up the antigen-binding site.
- Some parts of an antibody have unique functions. The arms of the Y for example, contain the sites that can bind two antigens (in general identical) and therefore recognize specific foreign objects. This region of the antibody is called the Fab (Fragment, antigen binding) region. It is composed of one constant and one variable domain from each heavy and light chain of the antibody.
- The variable domain is referred to as the FV region and is the most important region for binding to antigens.
- Fc region of the antibody is the region that triggers complement fixation reaction.

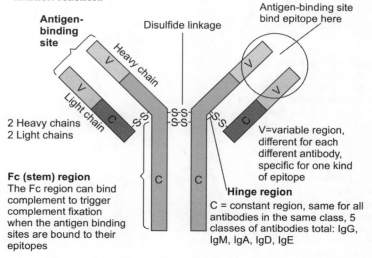

Figure 12.5: Basic structure of an antibody (immunoglobulin)

Classes of Antibodies/Immunoglobulins (Figure 12.6)

IgG Antibodies
• Monomer
• 80% of serum antibodies
• Produced on second+exposure
• In blood, lymph
• Can enter tissue, cross placenta
• Fix complement, enhance phagocytosis, neutralize toxin and viruses, protects fetus and newborn, antiserum

IgG

IgM Antibodies
• Pentamer
• 5–10% of serum antibodies
• Produced only on first exposure
• In blood, lymph, on B cells
• Fix complement, agglutinates antigen

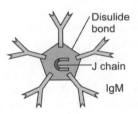

Disulide bond

J chain

IgM

IgA Antibodies
• Dimer
• 10–15% of serum antibodies
• In secretions
• Mucosal protection

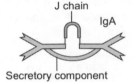

J chain

IgA

Secretory component

IgD Antibodies
• Monomer
• 0.2% of serum antibodies
• Surface receptor on B cells
• Initiate humoral immune response by B cells

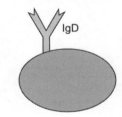

IgD

IgE Antibodies
• Monomer
• 0.002% of serum antibodies
• Surface receptor on mast cells and basophils
• Inflammation allergic reaction; lysis of parasitic worms

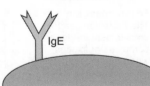

IgE

Figure 12.6: Classes of immunoglubulins

T-cells are the constituent of lymphocytes that undergo differentiation during immune respnse and develop into several sub-populations of effector T-cells that have an effect on many other cells. Some develop into T–Cytotoxic cells that attack and kill targets directly. Targets for Tc-cells include cells infected by viruses and cancerous cells. Other T-cells may develop into T-Helper cells and T-Supressor cells that stimulate the activities of other leukocytes through cell to cell contact or through secretion of cytokines. This part of immune response is called as Cellular or Cell-mediated immunity.

> The collaboration between B-cells and T-cells (Specially T-Helper cells) is important for almost all antibody responses to antigens.

Features of Adaptive Immunity (Figure 12.7)

- Specificity
  - Lymphocytes (B- and T-cells) bind and respond to foreign molecules (antigens) via antigen receptors: each to a specific antigen
- Diversity
  - The body possesses millions of lymphocytes that can recognise and respond to millions of antigens (one each)
- Memory
  - 1" exposure to an antigen generates lymphocytes and long-lived memory cells — next exposure to the same antigen, memory cells react more quickly and stronger response (acquired immunity')
- Self-Tolerance
  - Lymphocytes can distinguish self (our normal antigens) from non- sell (antigens from foreign material).

Table: 12.3: Difference between innate and adaptive immunity

Innate vs Adaptive Immunity	
Innate (Phagocyois, Inflammation)	Adaptive (Lymphocytes)
• Nonspecific Specific	• Specific
— Defends against *any* pathogen upon first exposure	— Responds to specific pathogens on 2nd or later exposure
— Responds to:	
• Infectious agents	— Comes into play after non specific responses have begun.
• Chemical irritants	
• Tissue injury	
• Burns	

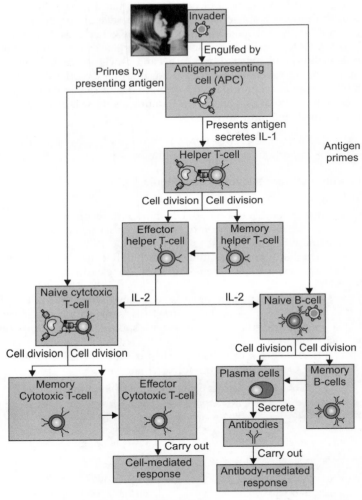

Figure 12.7: Summarizes an example of adaptive immune response when exposed to a microbial antigen

■ IMMUNIZATION (FIGURE 12.8)

Active and Passive Immunity

Adaptive immunity can either be active or passive, depending on whether the antibodies or T-cells are produced by the individual in response to antigens or are administered directly to the individual. Active Adaptive Immunity is produced by an individual either after natural exposure to antigens or after immunization. It is again of two types:

(i) Naturally acquired active immunity occurs when the person is exposed to a live pathogen, develops the disease and becomes immune as a result of the primary immune response.

(ii) Artificially acquired active immunity can be induced by a vaccine, a substance that contains the antigen. A vaccine stimulates a primary response against the antigen without causing symptoms of the disease. Passive adaptive immunity does not involve host's immune response at all. Rather, passive immunity occurs when preformed antibodies or T-cells are transferred from a donor to the recipient. It is also of two types:

(i) Naturally acquired passive immunity occurs during pregnancy in which certain antibodies are passed from the maternal into the fetal bloodstream.

(ii) Artificially acquired passive immunity can be induced when antibodies are injected into a pateint to fight against specific disease. For example: unvaccinated individuals, who are exposed to particular infectious agents often will be given preformed antibodies against those antigens. It is a short-term immunization by the injection of antibodies, such as Gamma Globulin (Ig G antibody), that are not produced by the recipient's cells.

■ VACCINES

A vaccine is a biological preparation that improves immunity to a particular disease. A vaccine typically contains an agent that resembles a disease-causing microorganism and is often made from weakened or killed forms of the microbe, its toxins or one of its surface proteins.

(a) Live Vaccines

The first live vaccine was cowpox virus introduced by Edward Jenner as a vaccine for Smallpox.

Live vaccines are used against a number of viral infections (Polio Sabin Vaccine), measles, mumps, rubella, chicken pox, hepatitis A, yellow fever, etc.). The only example of live bacterial vaccine is one against tuberculosis (*Mycobacterium bovis*: Bacille Calmette-Guerin vaccine: BCG). Live vaccines normally produce subsequent immunity, both humoral and cell-mediated.

Demerit of Live Vaccines

Since live vaccines are often attenuated (made less pathogenic) by passage in animals or thermal mutation, they can revert to their pathogenic form and cause serious illness. It is for this reason that live polio (Sabin) vaccine, which was used for many years, has been replaced in many countries by the inactivated (Salk) vaccine.

(b) Killed Vaccines

Killed (heat, chemical or UV irradiation) viral vaccines include those for Polio (Salk vaccine), Influenza, Rabies, etc. Most bacterial vaccines are killed organisms (Typhoid, Cholera, Plague, Pertussis, etc.)

(c) Subunit Vaccines

Subunit vaccines may consist of proteins or polysaccharides. Some antibacterial vaccines utilize purified cell wall components (*Hemophilus, Pertussis, Meningococcus, Pneumococcus*, etc.). Some viral vaccines (Hepatitis-B, etc.) consist of purified antigenic proteins manufactured after expression from a gene cloned into a suitable vector (e.g. yeast). When the pathogenic mechanism of an agent involves a toxin, a modified form of the toxin (toxoid, which has lost its toxicity while remaining immunogenic) is used as a vaccine (e.g. Diphtheria, Tetanus, Cholera).

Age	Birth	1	2	4	6	12	15	18	19-23	2-3	4-6
Vaccine						**Months**				**Years**	
Hepatitis-B1	HeB	HeB	1		HeB						HeB
Rotavirus			Rota	Rota	Rota						
Diphtheria, Tetanus, Pertussis			DTaP	DTaP	DTaP	3	DTaP				DTaP
Hemophilus influenzae-b (CV)[4]			Hib	Hib	Hib[4]	Hib					
Pncurnococcal[5]			PCV	PCV	PCV	PCV				PPV	
Inactivated Poliovirus			IPV	IPV	IPV						IPV
Influenza[6]					Influenza (Yearly)						
Measles, Mumps, Rubella[7]						MMR				MMR	MMR
Varicella[8]						Var					
Hepatitis A						Hep A (2 doses)			HepA series		
Meningococcal[10]									MCV4		

Figure12.8: Immunization schedule for normal children

Adverse Effects of Immunization

Active immunization may cause fever, malaise and discomfort. Some vaccine may also cause joint pains or arthritis (Rubella), convulsions, that may sometimes be fatal (Pertussis), or neurological disorders (Influenza). Allergies to eggs may develop as a consequence of viral vaccines produced in eggs (measles, mumps, influenza, yellow fever). The serious side effects have been documented after use of the DTP vaccine. Most of these were attributable to the whole pertussis component of the vaccine and have been eliminated by the use of an acellular pertussis preparation.

■ AUTOIMMUNITY (TABLE 12.4)

Our Immune system has the ability to tell the difference between self and nonself: what's you and what's foreign. If the immune system does not recognize its "self" it reacts against normal cells and tissues within the body. The body makes autoantibodies that attack normal cells by mistake. The result is misguided attack on your own body. This causes the damage we call it as autoimmune disaese or autoimmunity. There are more than 80 known types of autoimmunity.

Table: 12.4: Types of autoimmunity

Disease	Symptoms
Systemic lupus erythematosus (SLE)	Fever, arthritis, mouth ulcers, unusual loss of hair, swollen glands, chest pain, red rashes, etc
Rheumatoid arthritis (RA)	Inflammation and damage to the cartilage and bone of joints
Multiple Sclerosis (MS)	T-cells attack myelin present in muscle cells which results in blurred vision, muscle weakness, ataxia.
Autoimmune Hepatitis	Fatigue, enlarged liver, yellowing of skin, Itchy skin, Joint pain, stomach pain
Diabetes Type I (A disease in which own immune system attacks the cells that make insulin, a hormone to control blood sugar levels)	Being very thirsty, urinating often, feeling very hungry or tired, losing weight without trying, dry and itchy skin, tingling in the feet, blurry eyesight
Graves' Disease	Insomnia, irritability, weight loss, sweating, Muscle weakness, Bulging eyes, Shaky hands, light menstrual periods
Hemolytic Anaemia	Fatigue, shortness of breath, dizziness, headache, cold hands or feet, paleness, heart problems, etc.
Inflammatory Bowel Disease (IBD)	Abdominal pain, diarrhea (which may be bloody), fever, weight loss, fatigue, mouth ulcers, etc
Mysthenia Gravis (a disease in which the immune system attacks the nerves and muscles of the body)	Double vision, trouble in swallowing, weakness, drooping head, trouble climbing stairs, trouble talking

Cont...

Cont...

Disease	Symptoms
Scleroderma (A dieases causing abnormal growth of connective tissue in skin and blood vessels)	Fingers and toes turn white, pain and stiffness in fingers, fingers swollen, thickening of skin, tight facial skin, sores on fingers and toes, wight loss, trouble swallowing, diarrhea, etc.

▌ HYPERSENSITIVITY AND TYPES OF HYPERSENSITIVE REACTIONS (TABLE 12.5 TO 12.8)

Hypersensitivity refers to excessive undesirable (damaging, discomfort producing) reactions produced by normal immune system. Hypersesnsitivity requires a presensitized (immune) state of the host. Hypersensitivity reactions can be of 4 types: type I, type II, type III, type IV, based on the mechanisms involved and time taken for the reaction.

Type I Hypersensitivity

It is also known as immediate or anaphylactic hypersensitivity. The reaction may involve skin (eczema), eyes (conjunctivitis), nasopharynx (rhinitis), bronchopulmonary tissues (asthma) and gastrointestinal tract (gastroenteritis). The reaction takes 15-30 minutes from the time of exposure to the antigen. Sometimes, it is delayed to 10-12 hours.

Type I hypersensitivity is mediated by IgE. The primary cellular component in this hypersensitivity is mast cell or basophil. The reaction is amplified by platelets, neutrophils and eosinophils. The mechanism of reaction involves:

- Production of IgE in response to certain antigens often called as allergens
- IgE has very high affinity for its receptor (Fc; CD23) on mast cells and basophils.

A subsequent exposure of same allergen cross links the cell bound IgE and triggers the release of various pharmacologically active substances The agents released from mast cells and their effects are listed below:

Table 12.5: Pharmacologic mediators of immediate hypersensitivity

Mediator	Physiological effect
Preformed mediators in granules	
Histamine	Bronchoconstriction. mucus secretion. vasodialatation vascular permeability
Tryptase	Proteolysis

Cont...

Cont...

Mediator	Physiological effect
Kininogenase	Kinins and vasodialatation, vascular permeability, edema
ECF-A (teirapeptides)	Attract eosinophils and neutrophils
Leukotriene B_4	Basophil attractant
Leukotriene $C_4 D_4$	Similar to histamine but 1000 x more potent
Prosiaglandins D_2	Eosinophil and basophil chemotactic, histamine-like but more potent edema and pain
PAF	Platelet aggregation and heparin release: microthrombi

Diagnosis

Diagnostic tests for immediate hypersensitivity include:
- Skin (prick and intradermal) tests resulting in wheal and flare reaction, measurement of IgE and Specific IgE antibodies against the suspected allergens. It is done by an enzyme assay called as ELISA.

Treatment

- Symptomatic treatment is achieved with antihistamines that block histamine receptors
- Chromolyn sodium inhibits mast cell degranulation
- Late onset allergic symptoms such as bronchoconstriction which are mediated by leukotrienes are treated with leukotriene receptor blockers
- IgG antibodies against Fc portions of IgE that binds to mast cells has been approved for treatment of certain allergies, as it can block mast cell sensitization.

Anaphylaxis

Anaphylaxis is a severe, whole-body allergic reaction to a chemical that has become an allergen. After being exposed to a substance such as bee sting venom, the person's immune system becomes sensitized to it. When the person is exposed to that allergen again, an allergic reaction may occur. Anaphylaxis happens quickly after the exposure, is severe, and involves the whole body. Tissues in different parts of the body release histamine and other substances. This causes the airways to tighten and leads to other symptoms. Some drugs (morphine, X-ray dye, aspirin, and others) may cause an anaphylactic-like reaction (anaphylactoid reaction) when people are first exposed to them. Anaphylaxis can occur in response to any allergen. Common causes include:

- Drug Allergies
- Food Allergies
- Insect Bites/Sting

Symptoms develop quickly, often within seconds or minutes. They may include the following:

- Abdominal pain
- Abnormal (high-pitched) breathing sounds
- Anxiety
- Chest discomfort or tightness
- Cough
- Diarrhea
- Difficulty breathing
- Difficulty swallowing
- Dizziness or light-headedness
- Hives, itchiness
- Nasal congestion
- Nausea or vomiting
- Palpitations
- Skin redness
- Slurred speech
- Swelling of the face, eyes or tongue
- Unconsciousness
- Wheezing

Prevention

- Avoid triggers such as foods and medications that have caused an allergic reaction in the past. Ask detailed questions about ingredients when you are eating away from home. Also carefully examine ingredient labels.
- If you have a child who is allergic to certain foods, introduce one new food at a time in small amounts so you can recognize an allergic reaction.
- People who know that they have had serious allergic reactions should wear a medical ID tag.
- If you have a history of serious allergic reactions, carry emergency medications (such as a chewable form of diphenhydramine and injectable Epinephrine or a bee sting kit) according to your health care provider's instructions.
- Do not use your injectable epinephrine on anyone else. They may have a condition (such as a heart problem) that could be negatively affected by this drug.

Type II Hypersensitivity

It is also known as cytotoxic hypersensitivity and may affect a variety of organs and tissues. The antigens are normally endogenous, although exogenous chemicals that can attach to cell membranes can also lead to type II hypersensitivity. Drug induced Hemolytic anemia and Thrombocytopenia are such examples. The reaction time is minutes to hours. It is mediated primarily by antibodies of IgM or IgG class and complement. Phagocytes and Killer cells may also play a role.

Diagnosis

Diagnostic tests include detection of circulating antibody against tissues involved and the presence of antibody and complement in the lesion (biopsy) by immunoflorescence.

Treatment

It involves anti-inflammatory and immunosuppressive agents

Type III Hypersensitivity

It is also known as immune complex hypersensitivity. The reaction may be general (e.g. serum sickness) or may involve individual organs including skin (eg. systemic lupus erythromatosus), kidneys (e.g. lupus nephritis), lungs (e.g. aspergillosis), joints (e.g. rheumatoid arthritis) or other organs. This reaction may be pathogenic mechanism of diseases caused by many microorganisms. The reaction may take 3–10 hours after exposure to the antigen. It is mediated by soluble immune complexes and complement (C3a, 4a and 5a). They are mostly of IgG class, although IgM class also be involved. The antigen may be exogenous (bacterial, viral or parasitic infection) or endogenous (non-organ specific autoimmunity). The damage is caused by platelets and neutrophils.

Diagnosis

Diagnosis involves examination of tissue biopsies for deposits of Ig and complement by immunoflorescence. Presence of immune complexes in serum and depletion in complement level are also tested.

Treatment

It includes anti-inflammatory agents.

Type VI Hypersensitivity

It is also known as cell-mediated or delayed type hypersensitivity. The classical example of this type of hypersensitivity is tuberculin (Montoux) reaction that peaks 48 hours after the injection of antigen (tuberculin). The lesion is characterized by induration and Erythema. Type IV hypersensitivity is involved in the pathogenesis of many autoimmune and infectious diseases such as Tuberculosis, leprosy, etc.

Mechanism of damage in delayed hypersensitivity include T lymphocytes and monocytes and/or macrophages. The pathogenesis is triggered primarily by helper T-cells and secrete cytokines that activate and recruit macrophages, which cause the bulk of damage. The delayed hypersensitivity lesions mainly contain monocytes and T-cells. Major chemicals involved in this type of hypersensitivity include monocyte chemotactic factor, interleukin-2, interferon, TNF, etc.

Tablel 12.6: Delayed hypersensitivity reactions

Type	Reaction time	Clinical appearance	Histology	Antigen and site
Contact	48-72 hr	Eczema	Lymphocytes, followed by macrophages; edema of epidermis	Epidermal (organic chemicals, poison ivy, heavy metals, etc.)
Tuberculin	48-72 hr	Local induration	Lymphocytes, monocytes, macrophages	Intradermal (tuberculin, lepromin, etc.)
Granuloma	21-28 days	Hardening	Macrophages, epitheloid and giant cells, fibrosis	Persistent antigen or foreign body presence (tuberculosis, leprosy, etc.)

Table 12.7: Summary of hypersensitive reaction

Characteristics	Type-I (anaph lactic)	Type-II (cytotosic)	Type-III (cytotosic (immune complex)	Type-IV (delayed type)
Antibody	IgE	IgG, 1gM	IgG, 1gM	None
Antigen	Exogenous	Cell surface	Soluble	Tissues and organs
Response time	15-30 minutes	Minutes-hours	3-8 hours	48-72 hours
Appearance	Wheal and flare	Lysis and ne-crosis	Erythema and edema, necrosis	Erythema and induration
Histology	Basophils and eo-sinophil	Antibody and complement	Complement and neutro-phils	Macrophages and T-cells
Transferred with	Antibody	Antibody	Antibody	T-cells
Examples	Allergic asthma, hay fever	Erythroblastosis fetalis, Goodpas-ure's nephritis	SLE, farmer's lung disease	Tuberculin test, poison ivy granuloma

Table 12.8: Comparison of different types of hypersensitivity

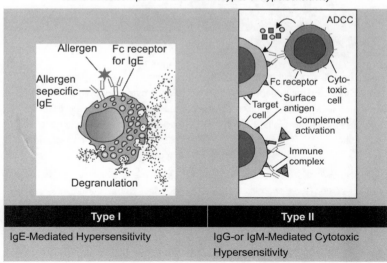

Type I	Type II
IgE-Mediated Hypersensitivity	IgG-or IgM-Mediated Cytotoxic Hypersensitivity

Cont...

Cont...

Ag induces cross-linking of IgE bound to mast cell and basophils with release of vasoactive mediators.	Ab directed against cell surface antigens mediates cell destruction via complement activation or ADCC.
Typical manifestations include systemic anaphylaxis and localized anaphylaxis such as hay fever, asthma, hives, food allergies, and eczema.	Typical manifestations include blood transfusion reactions, erythroblastosis fetalis, and autoimmune hemolytic anemia.

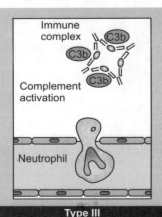 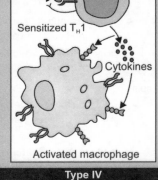

Type III	**Type IV**
Immune Complex-Mediated Hypersensitivity	Cell-Mediated Hypersensitivity
Ag-Ab complex deposited in various tissues induce complement activation and an ensuring inflammatory response mediated by massive infltration of neutrophils.	Sensitized TH1 cells shown above release cytokines that activate macrophages or TC cells that mediate direct cellular damage. TH2 cells and CTLs mediate similar responses.
Typical manifestations include localized arthus reaction and generalized recations such as serum sickness, necrotizing vasculitis, glomerulonephritis, rheumatoid arthritis, and systemic lupus erythematosus.	Typical manifestations include contact dermatitis, tubercular lesions, and graft rejection.

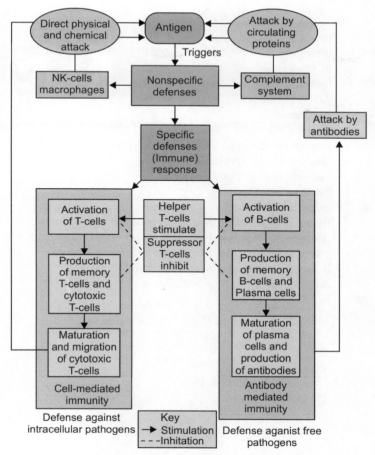

Figure 12.9: Summary of immune system

▮ POSSIBLE QUESTIONS:

1. Define immunity? Explain about active and passive immunity.
2. What is hypersensitivity? Explain the types of hypersensitivities.
3. Explain in detail the anaphylactic reaction and its preventive measures.
4. What is autoimmunity? Give a brief account of autoimmune diseases.

5. **Write Shorts Notes:**
   - Immunization Schedule
   - Immunity
   - BCG vaccine
   - Immunization
   - Active immunity
   - Vaccines
   - Anaphylaxis
   - Anaphylactic shock
   - Delayed type Hypersensitivity
   - Immediate Hypersensitivity
   - Rheumatoid Arthritis
6. **Differentiate between:**
   - Innate Immunity and Adaptive (acquired immunity)
   - Antigen and Antibody
   - T-cell and B-cell
   - Active immunity and passive immunity
   - Cell-mediated and humoral immunity

Chapter

13

Control and Destruction of Microorganisms

■ INTRODUCTION

The main reasons to control and destroy microorganisms are:
i.   to prevent transmission of disease and infection
ii. to prevent decomposition and spoilage
iii. to prevent contamination
This can be achieved by various ways.

■ IMPORTANT TERMS USED IN THE OF CONTROL MICROORGANISMS

Terms related to destruction of microorganisms are:

Sterilization : Destruction of all microorganisms, including endospores on an object or in a material.

Disinfection: The destruction of pathogens but not endospores on an object or in a material. The number of pathogens is reduced or growth is inhibited to a level that does not produce disease.

Antisepsis: Chemical disinfection of the skin, mucosal membranes or other living tissues.

Germicide ("cide" = kill) : A chemical agent that rapidly kills microorganisms. Specific germicides include:
- – Sporicide- kills spores
- – Bactericide- kills bacteria
- – Viricide- kills viruses
- – Fungicide- kills fungi

Chemotherapy: Chemicals used internally to kill or inhibit growth of microorganisms within host tissue.

Terms Related to Suppression of Microorganisms

i.   Asepsis: It means "without infection". It is the absence of pathogens from an object or area. Aseptic techniques prevent the entry of pathogens into the body.

There are two types of asepsis:

Surgical asepsis: Techniques designed to remove all microorganisms. It prevents infectious agents from reaching a wound.

Medical asepsis: Techniques designed to exclude microorganisms associated with communicable diseases. It includes dust control, hand-washing, use of individualized equipment and instruments, waste disposal, care of instruments, syringes, needles, thermometers and dressings.

ii.   Sanitization: The reduction or removal of pathogens on inanimate (non-living) objects by chemical or mechanical cleansing.

iii. Bacteriostasis: ("static" = halt) Bacterial growth and multiplication are inhibited, but the bacteria are not killed.

Terms for Destruction or Suppression of Microorganisms

- **Antimicrobial agents** – any substances that destroy or suppress microorganisms
- **Antibiotic** – a product formed by Microorganisms that destroy or suppress microorganism

■ PRINCIPLES OF MICROBIAL CONTROL

Methods used to control and destroy the growth of microorganisms and their transmission of infectious disease aim at:

- Stopping the growth of microorganism for a period of time
- Reducing the number of microorganisms to a safe level or
- Destroying the microorganisms

The degree of effectiveness of this process depends on following factors;

- Number of microorganisms
- Type of microorganism
- Their physiological state, such as the stage of growth or formation of endospores
- Environment in which they are growing (glassware, instruments, tissue, food).

The microorganisms can be controlled either by one or more of the following ways:

- Destroying the cell wall, or stopping the Cell wall synthesis.
- Destroy the Cell membrane.
- Denaturing (destroying the structure) protein and DNA.
- Stopping the protein synthesis.
- Stopping the DNA replication and transcription process.

■ METHODS OF MICROBIAL CONTROL

The methods of microbial control fall in one of the following categories;

- Disinfection
- Sterilization
- Antisepsis
- Chemotherapy

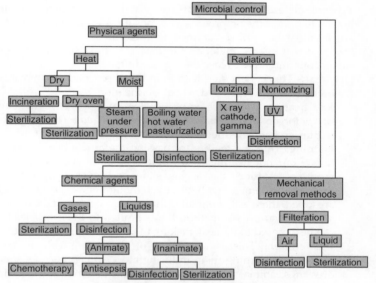

Figure 13.1: Microbiology control methods

Microbial control could be achieved by following ways:

- Physical Agents
- Chemical Agents
- Mechanical removal methods

Physical Agents

Heat

Heat is the most common, inexpensive, simplest, reliable and effective method used to destroy microorganisms. When heat is used for sterilization process in the presence of moisture then it is called as moist heat where as in the absence of moisture, it is called as dry heat.

i.   Basic Principle: Heat denatures (destroys the structure) Nucleic acids (DNA and RNA), proteins and enzymes of the microorganism. In absence of these molecules microorganisms can't survive.

ii.   Factors influencing sterilization by heat:

- Nature of heat: Moist heat is more effective than dry heat.

- Temperature and time: Temperature and time are inversely proportional. As temperature increases, the time taken is decreased.
- Number of microorganisms: More the number of microorganisms, higher the temperature or longer the duration required.
- Nature of microorganism: Depends on species and strain of microorganism, sensitivity to heat may vary. Spores are highly resistant to heat.
- Type of material: Articles that are heavily contaminated require higher temperature or prolonged exposure. Certain heat sensitive articles must be sterilized at lower temperature.
- Presence of Organic material: Organic materials such as protein, sugars, oils and fats increase the required time.
- **Dry heat -** This is heat sterilization in the absence of any moisture. Followings are the types of dry heat sterilization:
    - **Red heat:** Articles such as bacteriological loops, straight wires, tips of forceps and searing spatulas are sterilized by holding them in Bunsen flame till they become red hot.
    - **Flaming:** This is a method of passing the article over a Bunsen flame, but not heating it to redness. Articles such as scalpels, mouth of test tubes, flasks, glass slides and cover slips are passed through the flame a few times. Even though most vegetative cells are killed, there is no guarantee that spores too would die on such short exposure. This method too is limited to those articles that can be exposed to flame. Cracking of the glassware may occur.
    - **Incineration:** This is a method of destroying contaminated material by burning them in incinerator. Articles such as soiled dressings; animal carcasses, pathological material and bedding etc should be subjected to incineration. This technique results in the loss of the article, hence is suitable only for those articles that have to be disposed. Burning of polystyrene materials emits dense smoke and hence they should not be incinerated.
    - **Hot air oven:** This method was introduced by Louis Pasteur. Articles to be sterilized are exposed to high temperature (160°C) for duration of one hour in an electrically heated oven. Since air is poor conductor of heat, even distribution of heat throughout the chamber is achieved by a fan. The heat is transferred to the article by radiation, conduction and convection. The oven should be fitted with a thermostat control, temperature indicator, meshed shelves and must have adequate insulation.

Articles sterilized

Metallic instruments (like forceps, scalpels, scissors), glasswares (such as petri-dishes, pipettes, flasks, all-glass syringes), swabs, oils, grease, petroleum jelly and some pharmaceutical products.

Sterilization Process

Articles to be sterilized must be perfectly dry before placing them inside to avoid breakage. Articles must be placed at sufficient distance so as to allow free circulation of air in between. Mouths of flasks, test tubes and both ends of pipettes must be plugged with cotton wool. Articles such as petri dishes and pipettes may be arranged inside metal canisters and then placed. Individual glass articles must be wrapped in kraft paper or aluminum foils.

Advantages: It is an effective method of sterilization of heat stable articles. The articles remain dry after sterilization. This is the only method of sterilizing oils and powders.

Disadvantages:

- Since air is poor conductor of heat, hot air has poor penetration.
- Cotton wool and paper may get slightly charred.
- Glasses may become smoky.
- Takes longer time compared to autoclave.
    - **Infrared Rays:** Infrared rays bring about sterilization by generation of heat. Articles to be sterilized are placed in a moving conveyer belt and passed through a tunnel that is heated by infrared radiators to a temperature of 180°C. The articles are exposed to that temperature for a period of 7.5 minutes. Articles sterilized included metallic instruments and glassware. It is mainly used in central sterile supply department. It requires special equipments, hence is not applicable in diagnostic laboratory.
    - **Moist Heat:** This is heat sterilization in the presence of any moisture. Followings are the types of moist heat sterilization;

    At temperature below 100°C:
    - Pasteurization: This process was originally employed by Louis Pasteur. Currently this procedure is employed in food and dairy industry. There are two methods of pasteurization;
    - Holder method: Heated at 63°C for 30 minutes
    - Flash method: Heated at 72°C for 15 seconds followed by quickly cooling to 13°C
    - Ultra-High Temperature (UHT) Heated for 140°C for 15 sec and 149°C for 0.5 sec.

This method is suitable to destroy most milk borne pathogens like *Salmonella, Mycobacteria, Streptococci, Staphylococci* and *Brucella,* however *Coxiella* may survive pasteurization.

- **Vaccine bath:** The contaminating bacteria in a vaccine preparation can be inactivated by heating in a water bath at 60°C for one hour. Only vegetative bacteria are killed and spores survive.
- **Serum bath:** The contaminating bacteria in a serum preparation can be inactivated by heating in a water bath at 56°C for one hour on several successive days. Proteins in the serum will coagulate at higher temperature. Only vegetative bacteria are killed and spores survive.

At temperature 100°C:

– **Boiling:** Boiling water (100°C) kills most vegetative bacteria and viruses immediately. Certain bacterial toxins such as Staphylococcal enterotoxin are also heat resistant. Some bacterial spores are resistant to boiling and survive; hence this is not a substitute for sterilization.

Steam at 100°C: Instead of keeping the articles in boiling water, they are subjected to free steam at 100°C. A steamer is a metal cabinet with perforated trays to hold the articles and a conical lid. The bottom of steamer is filled with water and is heated. The steam that is generated sterilizes the articles when exposed for a period of 90 minutes. Media such as TCBS, DCA and selenite broth are sterilized by steaming.

At temperature above 100°C

– **Autoclave:** Sterilization can effectively be achieved at a temperature above 100°C using an Autoclave. Water boils at 100°C at atmospheric pressure, but if pressure is raised, the temperature at which the water boils also increases. In an autoclave the water is boiled in a closed chamber. As the pressure rises, the boiling point of water also raises. At a pressure of 15 lbs inside the autoclave, the temperature is said to be 121°C. Exposure of articles to this temperature for 15 minutes sterilizes them.

– **Advantages of Steam:** It has more penetrative power than dry air, it moistens the spores (moisture is essential for coagulation of proteins), condensation of steam on cooler surface releases latent heat, draws in fresh steam.

Construction and operation of Autoclave

- A simple Autoclave has vertical or horizontal cylindrical body with a heating element, a perforated tray to keep the articles, a lid that can be fastened by screw clamps, a pressure gauge, a safety valve and a discharge tap.
- The articles to be sterilized must not be tightly packed.
- The screw caps and cotton plugs must be loosely fitted.
- The lid is closed but the discharge tap is kept open and the water is heated. As the water starts boiling, the steam drives air out of the discharge tap.
- When all the air is displaced and steam start appearing through the discharge tap, the tap is closed.
- The pressure inside is allowed to rise upto 15 lbs per square inch. At this pressure the articles are held for 15 minutes, after which the heating is stopped and the Autoclave is allowed to cool.
- Once the pressure gauge shows the pressure equal to atmospheric pressure, the discharge tap is opened to let the air in.
- The lid is then opened and articles removed. Articles sterilized: Culture media, dressings, certain equipment, linen, etc.

Precautions

- Articles should not be tightly packed
- The Autoclave must not be overloaded
- Air discharge must be complete and there should not be any residual air trapped inside
- Caps of bottles and flasks should not be tight
- Autoclave must not be opened until the pressure has fallen or else the contents will boil over
- Articles must be wrapped in paper to prevent drenching, bottles must not be overfilled.

Advantage: Very effective way of sterilization, quicker than hot air oven.

Disadvantages: Drenching and wetting or articles may occur, trapped air may reduce the efficacy, takes long time to cool

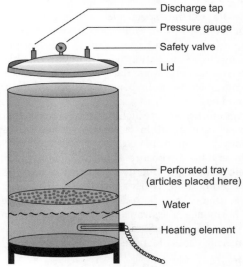

Figure 13.2: Autoclave

Radiation Sterilization

Two types of radiations are used, ionizing and non-ionizing. Non-ionizing rays are low energy rays with poor penetrative power while ionizing rays are high-energy rays with good penetrative power. Since radiation does not generate heat, it is termed "cold sterilization". In some parts of Europe, fruits and vegetables are irradiated to increase their shelf life up to 500 percent.

(a) Non-ionizing rays: Rays of wavelength longer than the visible light are non-ionizing. Microbicidal wavelength of Ultra violet-rays lie in the range of 200–280 nm with 260 nm being most effective. UV-rays are generated using a high-pressure mercury vapour lamp. Ultra violet-rays induce formation of Thymine-Thymine dimers, which ultimately inhibits DNA replication. Ultra Violet radiation readily induce mutations in cells irradiated with a non-lethal dose. Microorganisms such as bacteria, viruses, yeasts, etc. that are exposed to an effective UV-radiation are inactivated within seconds.

Disadvantages

- Low penetrative power of non-ionizing rays
- Limited life of the UV-bulb
- Some bacteria have DNA repair enzymes that can overcome damage caused by UV-rays
- Rays are harmful to skin and eyes
- It doesn't penetrate glass, paper or plastic

(b) Ionizing rays: Ionizing rays are of two types, particulate and electromagnetic rays.

- **Particulate Rays:** High speed electrons are produced by a linear accelerator from a heated cathode. Electron beams are employed to sterilize articles like syringes, gloves, dressing packs, foods and pharmaceuticals. Sterilization is accomplished in few seconds. Unlike electromagnetic rays, the instruments can be switched off. Disadvantage includes poor penetrative power and requirement of sophisticated equipment.
- **Electromagnetic rays:** These include Gamma rays which are produced from nuclear disintegration of certain radioactive isotopes (Co60, Cs137). They have more penetrative power than electron beam but require longer time of exposure. These high-energy radiations damage the Nucleic acid of the microorganism. A dosage of 2.5 megarads kills all bacteria, fungi, viruses and spores. It is used commercially to sterilize disposable petri-dishes, plastic syringes, antibiotics, vitamins, hormones, glasswares and fabrics. Disadvantages include; unlike electron beams, they can't be switched off, glasswares tend to become brownish, loss of tensile strength in fabric.

Chemical Methods

Disinfectants are those chemicals that destroy pathogenic bacteria from inanimate surfaces. Some chemical have very narrow spectrum of activity and some have very wide. Those chemicals that can sterilize are called chemisterilants. Those chemicals that can safely be applied over skin and mucus membranes are called antiseptics.

An ideal antiseptic or disinfectant should have following properties:

- Should have wide spectrum of activity
- Should be able to destroy microbes within practical period of time
- Should be active in the presence of Organic matter
- Should make effective contact and be wettable
- Should be active in any pH
- Should be stable

- Should have long shelf life
- Should be speedy
- Should have high penetrating power
- Should be non-toxic, non-allergenic, non-irritative or non-corrosive
- Should not have bad odour
- Should not leave non-volatile residue or stain
- Efficacy should not be lost on reasonable dilution
- Should not be expensive and must easily be available

Such an ideal disinfectant is not yet available.

Classification of disinfectants:

Based on consistency
- a. Liquid (e.g. Alcohols, Phenols)
- b. Gaseous (Formaldehyde vapour, Ethylene oxide)

Based on spectrum of activity
- a. High level
- b. Intermediate level
- c. Low level

Based on mechanism of action
- a. Action on membrane (e.g. Alcohol, detergent)
- b. Denaturation of cellular proteins (e.g. Alcohol, Phenol)

■ ALCOHOLS

- **Mode of action:** Alcohols dehydrate cells, disrupt membranes and cause coagulation of protein.
- **Examples:** Ethyl alcohol, Isopropyl alcohol and Methyl alcohol
- **Application:** A 70% aqueous solution is more effective at killing microbes than absolute alcohols. 70% Ethyl alcohol (spirit) is used as antiseptic on skin. Isopropyl alcohol is preferred to Ethanol. It can also be used to disinfect surfaces. It is used to disinfect clinical thermometers. Methyl alcohol kills fungal spores, hence is useful in disinfecting inoculation hoods.
- **Disadvantages:** Skin irritant, volatile (evaporates rapidly), inflammable.

■ ALDEHYDES

- **Mode of action** Acts through alkylation of amino-, carboxyl- or hydroxyl group, and probably damages Nucleic acids. It kills all Microorganisms, including spores.
- **Example** Formaldehyde, Gluteraldehyde
- **Application** 40% Formaldehyde (formalin) is used for surface disinfection and fumigation of rooms, chambers, operation theatres, biological safety cabinets, wards, sick rooms, etc.
- **Disadvantages** Vapours are irritating (must be neutralized by Ammonia), has poor penetration, leaves non-volatile residue, activity is reduced in the presence of protein. Gluteraldehyde requires alkaline pH and only those articles that are wettable can be sterilized.

◼ PHENOL

- **Mode of action:** Act by disruption of membranes, precipitation of proteins and inactivation of enzymes.
  Examples, 5% Phenol, 1-5% Cresol, 5% Lysol (a saponified cresol), Hexachlorophene, Chlorhexidine, Chloroxylenol (Dettol)
- **Applications:** Act as disinfectants at high concentration and as antiseptics at low concentrations. They are bactericidal, fungicidal, mycobactericidal but are inactive against spores and most viruses. They are not readily inactivated by organic matter. The corrosive phenolics are used for disinfection of ward floors, in discarding jars in laboratories and disinfection of bedpans.
- **Disadvantages:** It is toxic, corrosive and skin irritant. Chlorhexidine is inactivated by anionic soaps. Chloroxylenol is inactivated by hard water.

◼ HALOGENS

- **Mode of action:** They are Oxidizing agents and cause damage by oxidation of essential sulfydryl groups of enzymes. Chlorine reacts with water to form Hypochlorous acid which is microbicidal.
- **Examples:** Chlorine compounds (chlorine bleach, Hypochlorite) and iodine compounds (Tincture iodine, Iodophores)
- **Applications:** Chlorine gas is used to bleach water. Household bleach can be used to disinfect floors. 0.5% Sodium hypochlorite is used in Serology and Virology.
- **Disadvantages:** They are rapidly inactivated in the presence of Organic matter. Iodine is corrosive and staining. Bleach solution is corrosive and will corrode stainless steel surfaces.

◼ HEAVY METALS

- **Mode of action:** Act by precipitation of Proteins and oxidation of Sulfydryl groups. They are bacteriostatic.
  Examples: Mercuric chloride, Silver nitrate, Copper sulfate, Organic mercury salts (e.g., Mercurochrome, Merthiolate)
- **Applications:** 1% Silver nitrate solution can be applied on eyes as treatment for opthalmia neonatorum (Crede's method). Silver sulphadiazine is used topically to help to prevent colonization and infection of burn tissues.
- **Disadvantages:** Mercuric chloride is highly toxic are readily inactivated by Organic matter.

◼ SURFACE ACTIVE AGENTS

- **Mode of actions:** They have the property of concentrating at interfaces between lipid containing membrane of bacterial cell and surrounding aqueous medium. These compounds have long chain hydrocarbons that are fat soluble and charged ions that are water-soluble. Since they contain both of these, they concentrate on the surface of membranes. They disrupt membrane resulting in leakage of cell constituents.

- **Examples:** These are soaps or detergents.
- **Application:** They are active against vegetative cells, Mycobacteria and enveloped viruses. They are widely used as disinfectants at dilution of 1-2% for domestic use and in hospitals.
- **Disadvantages:** Their activity is reduced by hard water, anionic detergents and organic matter. *Pseudomonas* can metabolise cetrimide, using them as a carbon, nitrogen and energy source.

DYES

- **Mode of action:** Acridine dyes are bactericidal because of their interaction with bacterial nucleic acids.
  Examples: Aniline dyes such as Crystal violet, Malachite green and Brilliant green
- **Applications:** They may be used topically as antiseptics to treat mild burns. They are used as paint on the skin to treat bacterial skin infections. The dyes are used as selective agents in certain selective media.

HYDROGEN PEROXIDE

- **Mode of action:** It acts on Microorganisms through its release of nascent Oxygen. Hydrogen peroxide produces hydroxyl-free radical that damages proteins and DNA.
- **Application:** It is used at 6% concentration to decontaminate the instruments, equipments such as ventilators. 3% Hydrogen Peroxide Solution is used for skin disinfection and deodorising wounds and ulcers. Strong solutions are sporicidal.
- **Disadvantages:** Decomposes in light, broken down by Catalase, proteinaceous organic matter drastically reduces its activity.

ETHYLENE OXIDE (EO)

- **Mode of action:** It is an alkylating agent. It acts by alkylating sulfydryl-, amino-, carboxyl- and hydroxyl- groups.
- **Properties:** It is a cyclic molecule, which is a colorless liquid at room temperature. It has a sweet ethereal odour, readily polymerizes and is flammable.
- **Application:** It is a highly effective chemisterilant, capable of killing spores rapidly. Since it is highly flammable, it is usually combined with CO_2 (10% CO_2+ 90% EO) or DichloroDifluoroMethane. It requires presence of humidity.
- **Disadvantages:** It is highly toxic, irritating to eyes, skin, highly flammable, mutagenic and carcinogenic.

◼ BETA-PROPIOLACTONE (BPL)

- **Mode of action:** It is an alkylating agent and acts through alkylation of carboxyl- and hydroxyl- groups.
- **Properties:** It is a colorless liquid with pungent to slightly sweetish smell. It is a condensation product of ketone with formaldehyde.
- **Application:** It is an effective sporicidal agent and has broad-spectrum activity. 0.2% is used to sterilize biological products. It is more efficient in fumigation than Formaldehyde. It is used to sterilize vaccines, tissue grafts, surgical instruments and enzymes.
- **Disadvantages:** It has poor penetrating power and is a carcinogen.

Table 13.1: Common antiseptics and disinfectants

Chemical	Action	Uses
Ethanol (50–70%)	Denatures proteins and solubilizes lipids	Antiseptic used on skin
Isopropanol (50–70%)	Denatures proteins and solubilizes lipids	Antiseptic used on skin
Formaldehyde (8%)	Reacts with NH_2, SH and COOH groups	Disinfectant, kills endospores
Tincture of Iodine (2% I_2 in 70% alcohol)	Inactivates proteins	Antiseptic used on skin Disinfection of drinking water
Chlorine (Cl_2) gas	Forms hypochlorous acid (HClO), a strong oxidizing agent	Disinfect drinking water; general disinfectant
Silver nitrate ($AgNO_3$)	Precipitates proteins	General antiseptic and used in the eyes of new-borns
Mercuric chloride	Inactivates proteins by reacting with sulfide groups	Disinfectant, although occasionally used as an antiseptic on skin
Detergents (e.g. quaternary ammonium compounds)	Disrupts cell membranes	Skin antiseptics and disinfectants
Phenolic compounds (e.g. Carbolic acid, lysol, Hexylresorcinol, Hexachlorophene)	Denature proteins and disrupt cell membranes	Antiseptics at low concentrations; disinfectants at high concentrations
Ethylene oxide gas	Alkylating agent	Disinfectant used to sterilize heat-sensitive objects such as rubber and plastics
Ozone	Generates lethal oxygen radicals	Purification of water, sewage

■ CHEMOTHERAPY AND ANTIBIOTICS

Chemotherapeutic agents (synthetic antibiotics): antimicrobial agents of artificial origin are useful in the treatment of microbial or viral disease. Examples are Sulfonilamides, Isoniazid, Ethambutol, AZT, Nalidixic Acid and Chloramphenicol.

Antibiotics: Antimicrobial agents produced by microorganisms that kill or inhibit other microorganisms. Most clinically-useful antibiotics are produced by microorganisms and are used to kill or inhibit infectious Bacteria.

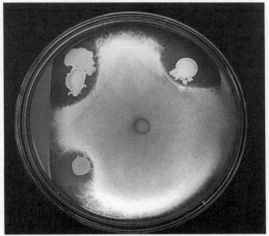

Figure 13.3: Three bacterial colonies growing on this plate secrete antibiotics that diffuse into the medium and inhibit the growth of a mold.

Properties of Antibiotics

- Antibiotics are low molecular-weight (non-protein) molecules produced as secondary metabolites, mainly by microorganisms that live in the soil.
- Most of these microorganisms form some type of a spore or other dormant cell and there is thought to be some relationship (besides temporal) between antibiotic production and the processes of sporulation.
- Among the molds, the notable antibiotic producers are *Penicillium* and *Cephalosporium* which are the main source of the beta-lactam antibiotics (Penicillin and its relatives).
- In the Bacteria, the Actinomycetes, notably *Streptomyces* species, produce a variety of types of antibiotics including the aminoglycosides (e.g. Streptomycin), Macrolides (e.g. Erythromycin), and the Tetracyclines. Endospore-forming Bacillus species produce polypeptide antibiotics

such as polymyxin and bacitracin. Table 13.2 is a summary of the classes of antibiotics, properties, biological sources, spectrum and mode of action.

Table 13.2: Classes of antibiotics and their properties

Chemical class	Examples	Biological source	Spectrum (effective against)	Mode of action
Beta-lactams (penicillins and cephalosporins)	Penicillin G, Cephalothin	*Penicillium notatum* and *Cephalosporium* species	Gram-positive bacteria	Inhibits steps in cell wall (peptidoglycan) synthesis and Murein assembly
Semi-synthetic penicillin	Ampicillin, Amoxycillin		Gram-positive and Gram-negative bacteria	Inhibits steps in cell wall (peptidoglycan) synthesis and murein assembly
Clavulanic Acid	Clavamox is clavulanic acid plus amoxycillin	*Streptomyces clavuligerus*	Gram-positive and Gram-negative bacteria	Suicide inhibitor of beta-lactamases
Monobactams	Aztreonam	*Chromobacter violaceum*	Gram-positive and Gram-negative bacteria	Inhibits steps in cell wall (peptidoglycan) synthesis and murein assembly
Carboxypenems	Imipenem	*Streptomyces cattleya*	Gram-positive and Gram-negative bacteria	Inhibits steps in cell wall (peptidoglycan) synthesis and murein assembly
Aminoglycosides	Streptomycin	*Streptomyces griseus*	Gram-positive and Gram-negative bacteria	Inhibit translation (protein synthesis)
	Gentamicin	*Micromonospora species*	Gram-positive and Gram-negative bacteria esp. *Pseudomonas*	Inhibit translation (protein synthesis)
Glycopeptides	Vancomycin	*Streptomyces orientales*	Gram-positive bacteria, esp. *Staphylococcus aureus*	Inhibits steps in murein (peptidoglycan) biosynthesis and assembly

Cont...

Cont...

Chemical class	Examples	Biological source	Spectrum (effective against)	Mode of action
Lincomycins	Clindamycin	*Streptomyces lincolnensis*	Gram-positive and Gram-negative bacteria esp. anaerobic Bacteroides	Inhibits translation (protein synthesis)
Macrolides	Erythromycin	*Streptomyces erythreus*	Gram-positive bacteria, Gram-negative bacteria not enterics, *Neisseria, Legionella, Mycoplasma*	Inhibits translation (protein synthesis)
Polypeptides	Polymyxin	*Bacillus polymyxa*	Gram-negative bacteria	Damages cytoplasmic membranes
	Bacitracin	*Bacillus subtilis*	Gram-positive bacteria	Inhibits steps in murein (peptidoglycan) biosynthesis and assembly
Polyenes	Amphotericin	*Streptomyces nodosus*	Fungi	Inactivate membranes containing sterols
	Nystatin	*Streptomyces noursei*	Fungi (Candida)	Inactivate membranes containing sterols
Rifamycins	Rifampicin	*Streptomyces mediterranei*	Gram-positive and Gram-negative bacteria, *Mycobacterium tuberculosis*	Inhibits transcription (eubacterial RNA polymerase)
Tetracyclines	Tetracycline	*Streptomyces species*	Gram-positive and Gram-negative bacteria, Rickettsias	Inhibit translation (protein synthesis)
Semisynthetic tetracycline	Doxycycline		Gram-positive and Gram-negative bacteria, *Rickettsias Ehrlichia, Borrelia*	Inhibit translation (protein synthesis)
Chloramphenicol	Chloramphenicol	*Streptomyces venezuelae*	Gram-positive and Gram-negative bacteria	Inhibits translation (protein synthesis)

■ ASEPSIS (FIGURE : 13.4)

Asepsis is the state of being free from disease-causing contaminants (such as bacteria, viruses, fungi, and parasites) or preventing contact with microorganisms. The term **asepsis** often refers to those practices used to promote or induce asepsis in surgery or medicine to prevent infection.
Asepsis is divided into the following two categories:

I.   Medical asepsis consists of techniques that inhibit the growth and spread of pathogenic microorganisms. Medical asepsis is also known as clean technique and is used in many daily activities, such as hand hygiene and changing patients' bed linen. Principles of medical asepsis can be followed in the home, for instance, with the common practice of washing your hands before preparing food.
Following are the principles of Medical asepsis:

Handwashing – Handwashing is the single most important means of preventing the spread of infection in the hospital. Hands should be washed.

- Before beginning work
- After using the bathroom
- Before and after patient contact
- Before eating and leaving work

Using mechanical friction, all areas of the arms, lower than the elbows, should be well lathered and scrubbed. Special attention should be given to the nails and nail beds. Rings and jewelry should be removed from hands and wrists because these articles may shelter large numbers of microorganisms. Thoroughly rinse hands under running water.

Dressing Changes – Wash hands and use gloves as necessary. Remove dressings using no-touch technique and place them in a disposable bag. The physician will remove the sutures. Place the removed sutures in the disposable bag. If needed, apply a sterile dressing. Never touch the skin around a wound without sterile gloves being worn. Place tightly closed disposable bag in the infectious waste receptacle in soiled utility room. Wash hands. The use of gloves does not negate the importance of hand washing before and after patient care.

Preoperative Shave procedure – The purpose of preoperative shave is to cleanse, to remove hair from the operative site. It is important to be informed of the exact area to be prepared for any out of the ordinary aspects, i.e., rashes, lesions, warts or other skin eruptions. Nicking the skin during prepping increases the possibility of infection. Report any of these observations to your supervisor and the physician before continuing with the prep. If the skin is nicked, an Incident report shall be completed. The physician shall be notified immediately. The pre-operative preparation should be done as close to the time of surgery as practical as feasible. At times, clipping of hair or a depilatory agent will be used instead of shaving. This is also an acceptable practice.

Urinary Catheter – Scrupulous aseptic technique in catheter insertion and daily cleaning at the point of insertion of the catheter with soap and water is utilized to reduce the incidence of infection.

Emptying Urinary Catheter Bags – When a care provider is emptying a urinary catheter bag, this should be viewed as a single interaction for a single patient and the tasks for one patient should be completed before going to the next patient. Wearing gloves for emptying catheter bags is wise because it is difficult not to get urine on the hands. It is unacceptable to consider it a single task to empty the catheter bags for several patients in sequence without changing gloves and washing hands between patients. This is because of the real risk of transmitting organisms from the catheter bag drainage spout of one patient to the next patient's drainage spout on the hands of personnel.

Intravenous – Aseptic technique is mandatory in the preparation and administration of intravenous solutions. The longer the catheter remains in place, the greater the potential of infectious complications.

Care of the Body after Death from Infectious Disease – Infection control is of prime importance in the care of the body after death when the deceased patient has had an infectious disease. When taking care of a deceased patient who has had an airborne infectious disease, prescribed isolation technique should be followed and the patient's body labeled with "Airborne Precautions" before being transported to the morgue. All other patients are cared for under Standard Precautions Policy and Procedures .

Personal Hygiene – All hospital personnel must be hygienic. If any employee is hygienically offensive, it is your responsibility to report the situation to the proper supervisor.

Employee Rashes or Skin Lesions – Lesions on body such as boils, abscesses, impetigo, etc., must be reported to the employee's supervisor. The employee shall be referred to Occupational health

Patients with Rashes or Skin Lesions – The most important intervention for rashes or skin lesions is to call it to the attention of the patient's physician and determine its cause promptly. In many cases, prompt recognition of the rash, identification of the cause, and prompt appropriate intervention can prevent transmission to the care provider and others. If a transmissible skin condition is identified, a "CONTACT PRECAUTIONS" sign shall be placed on the door of the patient's room so that ALL personnel can be advised of the protective barriers to be utilized.

Skin Punctures/Blood and Body Fluid Exposure – If you break skin from a sharp object or sustain a blood or body fluid splash to the eyes, nose, or mouth or to open areas of your skin, you are required to report the incident to your supervisor for referral to Occupational Health Services. An Incident Report is to be completed.

Equipment Handling – Equipment used for patient care is contaminated after use whether visible soiled or not. Reusable equipment must be cleaned and disinfected before being used for another patient. Hands must be washed immediately after use of equipment for patient care.

Sterilized Articles – Articles which have been sterilized must be carefully protected from contamination. Initial and expiration date shall be put on all packs and containers of sterile articles. If articles are not used within the specified period of time or if the packs become wet or damaged, the articles must be sterilized again. Consider all opened, wet or damaged packs as contaminated.

Work Area Sanitation – Work areas must be free from refuse, especially around refuse disposal units. Refuse in high risk areas – Surgical Suites, Laboratory, Dietary, Emergency room, Isolation rooms and central sterile processing should be removed at least twice during the day shift.

Disposable Equipment and Supplies – Disposable equipment and supplies should be used whenever possible. Some of the used supplies become infectious waste if contaminated with large amounts of blood or body fluids or after use in high-risk areas.

Handling of All Specimens – All specimens of blood or body fluids such as sputum, feces, urine or drainage from anybody site should be handled as if it were a source of infection. Disposable specimen containers are to be used and their disposal must be proper. Caution should be taken by persons who collect, transport and test specimens in order to prevent transmission of infection. All specimens should be transported to the laboratory in specimen transport bags.

Storage of Clean Equipment – All IV poles, weight scales, walkers, etc. should be stored in a clean storage area. These items should be wiped down with a disinfectant after patient use before storage.

Needle Syringe Disposal – Used needles and syringes are potential health hazards and should be treated with care. Contaminated needles and syringes must be discarded uncapped and unbroken into a needle and other sharps disposal boxes. Needle disposal boxes, when full, will be removed by Building Services.

Food – Food products are a major source of infectious microorganisms. The consumption of food by employees is forbidden in patient and/or work areas. Employees have designated areas for food consumption.

Various warm – Blooded animals are recognized as reservoirs of infectious disease agents of man. Because of this zoonosis, warm-blooded animals are forbidden in the hospital. A seeing-eye dog may be accompanied by a legally blind individual to certain areas of the hospital. Administrative policy may be seen. If rodents are observed, it is the responsibility of employee to report the incident to a supervisor.

Insects – Insects such as flies, cockroaches, etc. are main source for transmitting disease. All employees are to be instructed to report to their supervisor or any member of the Infection Control Committee when insects are observed.

Warning Signs – All warning signs such as Biohazard, Isolation Precautions, Do Not Enter, Radioactivity, etc. are to be recognized and observed by all employees.

Refrigerators – Food is not to be stored in refrigerators containing medications, blood products, biohazard specimens or chemicals.

Smoking – Cigarettes are not sold in the hospital. Smoking is not allowed inside the hospital.

Preparation of Medication Sites – All patient skin sites utilized for intradermal, subcutaneous or intramuscular injections are to be cleaned prior to injecting with a disinfectant such as alcohol suitable for topical use. All intravenous injection ports are likewise to be cleaned prior to and after manipulation with alco-wipes.

II. **Surgical asepsis** destroys all microorganisms and their **spores** (the reproductive cells of some microorganisms, such as fungi or protozoa). Surgical asepsis is known as sterile technique and is used in specialized areas or skills, such as care of surgical wounds, urinary catheter insertion, invasive procedures and surgery.

Principles and practices of surgical asepsis.

Start with sterile equipment and set-up the sterile field.

- All objects used in a sterile field must be sterile.
- Confirm sterility of the package. – Check expiration date and ensure package is clean and dry.
- Open the package – Place in centre of table; top flap open away from you; touch only outside of wrapper; side flaps open with each hand; 4th flap towards you making sure it does not touch your uniform. If the inner surface touches any unsterile article it is contaminated.
- Opening a wrapped package while holding it: same as above.
- Using a drape to establish a field; with one hand pluck the corner of the drape that is folded back on the top.
    - Lift the drape out of the cover and allow it to open freely without touching any objects.
    - Lay the drape on a clean dry surface, placing the freely hanging side farthest from you (nurse should not lean over sterile field).
- If there is any doubt about the sterility of an object consider it unsterile, e.g. the package falls on the floor or has evidence of damage or moisture, even dried moisture.

Maintain the Sterile field from Start to Finish.

- The skin cannot be sterilized and is unsterile.
- Sterile persons and items contact only sterile areas, unsterile persons and items contact only unsterile areas.
- Sterile objects become unsterile when touched by unsterile objects.
- Sterile objects can become unsterile by prolonged exposure to airborne microorganisms. Do not cough, sneeze or talk excessively over a sterile field.

- Use a sterile package immediately once it has been opened. Leftover sterile solutions are no longer sterile and should be discarded.
- Sterile items that are out of vision or below the waist level of the Nurse are considered unsterile. Sterile areas are continuously kept in view.
- Always face a sterile field. If you turn your back on a sterile field, you cannot guarantee its sterility.
- Movement within and around a sterile field must be such as not to cause contamination of that sterile field.
- Fluids flow in the direction of gravity. Moisture that passes through a sterile object draws microorganisms from unsterile surfaces above or below to the sterile surface by capillary action.
- The edges of sterile containers are not considered sterile once the package is open. The one inch margin around the edge of the sterile field is considered contaminated.
- Sterile gowns are considered sterile in front, shoulder to table level. The sleeves are also sterile.
- Tables are sterile only at table top level.
- Whenever bacterial barriers are permeated, contamination occur.
- Articles of doubtful sterility are considered unsterile.
- Conscientiousness, alertness and honesty are essential qualities in maintaining surgical asepsis.

Sterile Supplies

- Open each wrapped package as described above
- With free hand, grasp the corners of the wrapper and hold them against the wrist of the other hand (the unsterile hand is now covered by the sterile wrapper).
- Place the sterile item on the field by approaching from an angle rather than holding the arm over the field.
- Commercially packaged supplies: Hold the package above the field and allow contents to drop on centre of the field.
- Sterile solutions: Read label to confirm solution. Outside of container is unsterile; inside sterile. Once it is opened, its sterility cannot be ensured for future use. Remove cap and inert before placing it on a table. Hold the bottle of fluid at a height of about 4-6" and to the side of the sterile field; discard a little solution before pouring; avoid splashing which will cause the field to be contaminated.
- Use of sterile forceps: Keep the tips of wet forceps lower than the wrist at all times. Hold sterile forceps above waist level and in sight.
- Sterile Gloves- May be donned by open or closed method. Closed method requires a sterile gown so in the general care area, the open method is used. Gloves may be latex or vinyl and come in sizes.

The Surgical Team

- Team members are categorized as sterile or nonsterile in relation to the sterile surgical field.

- Sterile team members are those who scrub their hands and arms, don sterile attire, use sterile instruments and supplies and work in the sterile surgical field. This includes the surgeon, physician assistant and RN first assistant and the scrub person who may be a RN, a LVN or a surgical technician.
- The RNFA (Registered Nurse First Assistant) replaces an assisting surgeon and has had additional training. The duties include handling tissue and organs with instruments, providing exposure of the surgical site, suturing, etc.
- The scrub nurse (or surgical scrub technician) sets up and maintains the sterile field, hands supplies and instruments to the surgeon, keeps accurate count of instruments, sponges sharps and monitors aseptic technique.
- Nonsterile team members have responsibilities outside the sterile field and do not wear sterile attire.
    - The nonsterile team members include the anaesthesiologists, the nurse anaesthetist, and the circulating nurse.
    - The circulating nurse must be an RN and she coordinates the care of the client and manages activities outside the sterile field.

Medical Asepsis	Surgical Asepsis

– Reduces number of pathogens
– Referred to as
  "Clean teciniques"
– Uset administration of:
• Medications
• Enemas
• Tube feedings
• Daily hygiene
• Handwshing is number
• Mepical Asepsis
	– Eliminats all pathogens
	– Refered to as
	  "Sterile technique"
	– Used in:
	• Dressing changes
	• Cheterizations
	• Surgical Procedures
	• Surgical Asepsis

Figure 13.4: Medical asepsis and surgical asepsis

■ PRACTICAL PROCEDURES FOR HANDWASHING (FIGURES 13.5 (1 TO 12))

Effective hand washing procedures can remove all transient bacteria. The adoption of this simple but effective technique has been demonstrated to significantly reduce rates of hospital acquired infection.

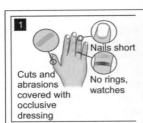

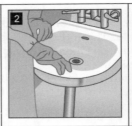

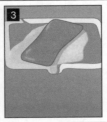

Some general points need emphasising: Keep nails short; avoid wearing rings and watches; cover cuts and cterproof dressings to reduce the risk of blood-borne infection such as hepatitis B, C and HIV.	Hands should be decontaminated even if gloves have been worn – they may be punctured or leak. Even if the gloves are intact, hands can become contaminated as the gloves are removed. A Sink with elbow or foot-operated taps should be used if at all possible.	Dispensers for soaps and skin disinfectants should be designed to prevent contaminate of the contents when they are handled. Bars of soap become contaminated easily and contribute to the risks of cross-infection.

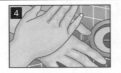

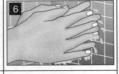

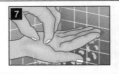

Effective decontamination technique starts with dispensing soap or skin disinfectant onto the moistened hands. Rub the palms together vigorously to aid the removal of dead cells and bacteria.	Ensure hand surfaces receive contact. It helps to have a set routine – always decontaminate the dorsal surface after the palms.	Remember to decontaminate the inter digital spaces as they are often heavily contaminated.

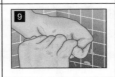

Decontaminate the fingertips of each hand in turn to create friction against the palm of the opposing hand.	Clasp the hands together, ensuring that thumbs and wrists receive contact with each other.	Avoid splashing during the hand decontamination routine so as to avoid contaminating clothing and the surrounding environment.

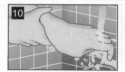	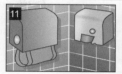	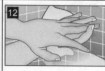
Rinse all hand surface thoroughly: residual soap or antiseptic can make the skin sore and dry. After thorough rinsing turn the tap off by the elbow or feet. Take care not to recontaminate the hands by touching the tap.	As wet surface transfter microorganisms more effectively than dry ones, always dry the hands thoroughly with a paper towel. Communal towels promote cross-infection, while driers circulate air loaded with bacteria.	Friction caused by the hands on the paper towel helps to remove remaining bacteria. In the community. It may be necessary to carry paper towels to homes where hand decontamina-tion facilities are in-adequate.

Figures 13.5 (1 to 12): Technique of handwashing

■ CROSS INFECTION

Cross infection is the transfer of harmful Microorganisms. Bacteria and Viruses are among the most common. The spread of infections can occur between people, pieces of equipment or within the body. These infections can cause many complications. Medical professionals work diligently to ensure equipment safety and a clean environment.

Types of Cross Infection

Cross infection can stem from:
- Bacteria
- Fungi
- Parasites
- Viruses

Causes of Cross Infection

Cross infections are caused by:
- Unsterilized medical equipment
- Bacteria from coughing and sneezing
- The transmission of viruses through human contact
- Touching contaminated objects
- Dirty bedding

Symptoms of Cross Infection

The exact symptoms of cross infection depend on the source. For example, an infection caused by a catheter can result in a Urinary Tract Infection

(UTI). The symptoms include pain in the kidneys, abdomen and groin. Infections spread through surgery may cause redness, swelling, and pus at the operation site. One of the first telling signs of a cross infection is a fever. This is usually the body's first course of action to help to get rid of an infection.

Diagnosing Cross Infection

Doctors may use a combination of methods to diagnose cross infection. These include:
- Physical examination
- Blood tests
- Culture tests
- Urine tests
- X-rays
- Health history review

Treating Cross Infection

Treating cross infection depends on the condition. Antibiotics are often used for bacterial infections. These medicines don't treat viruses. The problem with antibiotics is that bacteria can learn to adapt and potentially become resistant to medications overtime. This not only leads to individual resistance, but can lead to the evolution of "superbugs." These are strains of bacteria immune to antibiotics, which make the risk for related complications high.

Prescription of anti-viral drugs are used to treat specific types of viruses. Anti-fungal medications can be used to treat fungal infections, either in topical or oral form. Parasites transferred through cross infection may be treated with antibiotics as well as dietary changes.

Cross Infection Complications

Untreated bacterial and viral infections can lead to:
- Diarrhoea
- Pneumonia
- Meningitis
- Death

Preventing Cross Infection

Cross infection is the best treated at the source. Medical professionals use techniques to help preventing infections at facilities as well as during and after surgical procedures. Aseptic technique is a common process used to properly sterilize equipment so that harmful microorganisms can't spread from patient to patient.

■ CONTROL OF SPREAD OF INFECTION

Infection Control in a Health Care Facility is the prevention of spreading of microorganisms from:

- Patient to patient
- Patient to hospital Staff member
- Hospital Staff member to patient

Who does Infection Control?

Every Health care facility should have a nominated person or team to ensure Infection Control Policies and Procedures are in place. However, all employees who have contact with patients or items used in the care of patients must adhere to Infection Control Policies and Procedures.

Why is Infection Controls important in Health care facilities?

In most Health care facilities many sick people are treated or cared for in confined spaces. This means there are many microorganisms present. Patients will come into contact with many members of staff who can potentially spread the microorganisms and infections between patients. Large amounts of waste contaminated with blood and body substances are handled and processed in Health care settings increasing the risk of infection.

The following Medical procedures also increase the risk of infection:

- Inserting a tube into the body to drain or deliver fluids provides a pathway through which bacteria can enter.
- Surgery requires cutting the skin which is one of the body's most important defences against infection.
- The over-use of Antibiotics have caused the development of some drug resistant bacteria that are harder to destroy. Controlling the spread of infections in a health care facility is, therefore, very important.

Note that the risk of people working in health care facilities getting infections from patients is very low if all staff members follow good hygiene principles and other Standard Precautions.

General Infection Control Measures

Implementation and adherence to infection control practices are the keys to prevent transmission of healthcare associated infections including respiratory diseases spread by droplet or airborne routes. Recommended infection control practices include the following:

- Hand hygiene
- Standard precautions/transmission-based precautions (Contact, Droplet, Airborne) and
- Respiratory hygiene
- **Hand Hygiene**

Proper hand hygiene is the most effective way to prevent the spread of infection.

- Wash hands with soap and water when they are visibly dirty or soiled with blood or other body fluids.
  - When washing hands with soap and water, wet hands with water, apply soap to hands and rub them together vigorously for at least 15 seconds covering all surfaces of the hands and fingers.
  - Rinse hands with water and dry thoroughly with a disposable towel. Use towel to turn off the faucet.
- If hands are not visibly soiled, an alcohol-based hand rub or gel may be used in place of soap and water.
  - When using an alcohol-based hand rub or gel, apply product to the palm of one hand and rub hands together covering all surfaces of hands and fingers until the hands are dry.
  - Avoid wearing artificial fingernails when caring for patients at high risk for infection and keep natural nail tips less than 1/4-inch long.
  - Wear gloves when contact with blood, mucous membranes, non intact skin or other potentially infectious materials could occur.
  - Remove gloves after caring for a patient. Always perform hand hygiene after removing gloves. Never wear the same pair of gloves for the care of more than one patient.
  - Change gloves during patient care if moving from a contaminated body site to a clean body site.

Standard Precautions

Standard precautions and transmission-based precautions are designed to prevent transmission of infectious microorganisms. They require the use of work practice controls and protective apparel for all contacts with blood and body substances and airborne infection isolation, droplet and contact precautions for patients with diseases known to be transmitted in whole or in part by those routes. Standard precautions include consistent and prudent preventive measures to be used at all times, regardless of a patient's infection status.

Standard precautions include the following:

Hand hygiene Practice hand hygiene after touching blood, body fluids, secretions, excretions or contaminated items, whether or not gloves are worn. Wash hands immediately after gloves are removed between patient contacts and when otherwise indicated to avoid transfer of microorganisms to other patients or environment.

Gloves Wear gloves (clean, nonsterile gloves are adequate) when touching blood, body fluids, secretion, excretion, or contaminated items. Put on clean gloves just before touching mucous membranes and nonintact skin.

Change gloves between tasks and procedures. Practice hand hygiene whenever gloves are removed.

Mask, eye protection/face shield. Wear a mask and adequate eye protection (eyeglasses are not acceptable), or a face shield to protect mucous membranes of the eyes, nose and mouth during procedures and patient care activities that are likely to generate splashes or sprays of blood, body fluids, secretion, or excretion.

Gown Wear a gown (a clean, nonsterile gown is adequate) to protect skin and to prevent soiling of clothing during procedure and patient care activities that are likely to generate splashes or sprays of blood, body fluids, secretion or excretion. Remove a soiled gown as promptly as possible, with care to avoid contamination of clothing, and wash hands.

Patient care Equipment. Handle used patient care equipment soiled with blood, body fluids, secretion, or excretion in a manner that prevents skin and mucous membrane exposures, contamination of clothing and transfer of microorganisms to one's self, other patients and environment. Ensure that reusable equipment is not used for the care of another patient until it has been cleaned and sanitized appropriately. Ensure that single-used items are discarded properly.

Droplet Precautions

In addition to standard precautions, use droplet precautions for a patient known or suspected to be infected with microorganisms transmitted by droplets (large-particle, wet droplets [larger than 5mµ in size]) that can be generated by the patient during coughing, sneezing, talking or in the course of procedure.

Droplet precautions include the following:

Patient placement: Place the patient in a private room. When a private room is not available, place the patient in a room with a patient who has active infection with the same microorganism but with no other infection (cohorting). When a private room is not available and cohorting is not achievable, maintain spatial separation of at least six feet between the infected patient and other patients and visitors. Special air handling and ventilation are not necessary and the door may remain open.

Mask: In addition to standard precautions, wear a mask or respirator when working within three to six feet of the patient. (Hospitals may want to implement the practice of wearing a mask to enter the room.)

Patient transport: Limit the movement and transport of the patient from the room to essential purposes only. If transport or movement is necessary, minimize patient dispersal of droplets by masking the patient, if possible.

Contact Precautions

In addition to standard precautions, contact precautions should be used for the care of patients known or suspected to have illnesses that can be spread by usual contact with an infected person or the surfaces or patient care items in the room.

Contact precautions include the following:

- **Gloves and hand hygiene**: Wear gloves when entering the room. During the course of providing care for a patient, change gloves after having contact with infectious material. Remove gloves before leaving the patient's room and wash hands immediately with an antimicrobial agent or use a waterless antiseptic agent. After glove removal and hand washing, ensure that hands do not touch potentially contaminated surfaces or items in the patient's room.
- **Gown**: Wear a gown when entering the room. Remove the gown before leaving the patient's environment. After gown removal, ensure that clothing does not contact potentially contaminated environmental surfaces. Wash or decontaminate hands.
- **Patient transport**: Limit the movement of the patient from the room to essential purposes only. During transport, ensure that all precautions are maintained.
- **Patient care equipment**: When possible, dedicate the use of noncritical patient care equipment to a single patient (or cohort of patients infected or colonized with the pathogen requiring precautions) to avoid sharing between patients. If use of common equipment or items is unavoidable, then adequately clean and disinfect them before use for another patient.
- **Patient placement (private room)**: Place the patient in a private room. If a private room is not available, place the patient in a room with other patients with the same illness (cohorting). Apply appropriate cleaning and decontamination of the room after the patient has vacated it.

Airborne Infection Isolation

In addition to standard precautions, airborne infection isolation measures are designed to reduce the risk of transmission of infectious microorganisms that may be suspended in the air either in small particle aerosols or dust. Patients requiring airborne infection isolation must be given a private room with special air handling and ventilation (negative pressure). Respiratory protection for Healthcare workers is necessary when entering the patient's room.

Respiratory Hygiene/Cough Etiquette

"Respiratory hygiene" includes the measures that can be taken to decrease the risk of spreading respiratory pathogens. A universal "respiratory hygiene/cough etiquette" strategy for a healthcare facility should include the following:

- Place signs at the entrances of all outpatient facilities requesting that patients and visitors inform healthcare personnel of respiratory symptoms upon registration.
- Provide masks (e.g., surgical) for all patients presenting with respiratory symptoms (especially cough) and provide instructions on the proper use and disposal of masks.
- If a patient cannot wear a mask, provide tissues and instructions on when to use them (i.e., when coughing, sneezing or controlling nasal secretions), how and where to dispose of them and the importance of hand hygiene after handling this material
- Provide hand hygiene materials in waiting room areas and encourage patients with respiratory symptoms to wash their hands
- If possible, designate an area in waiting rooms where patients with respiratory symptoms can be segregated (ideally by more than three feet) from other patients without respiratory symptoms
- Place patients with respiratory symptoms in a private room or cubicle as soon as possible for further evaluation.
- Healthcare workers evaluating patients with respiratory symptoms should wear a surgical or procedure mask.
- Consider the installation of Plexiglas barriers at the point of triage or registration to protect Healthcare workers.
- If a physical barrier is not possible, instruct registration and triage staff to remain at least three to six feet from unmasked patients. Staff should consider wearing a surgical mask during registration and triage.
- Continue to use droplet precautions to manage patients with respiratory symptoms until it is determined that the cause of symptoms is not an infectious agent that requires precautions beyond standard precautions.

■ POSSIBLE QUESTIONS

1. Define sterilization and explain briefly the methods of sterilization.
2. What are the roles of nurses in preventing cross infections?
3. Give a detail account of chemical agents used for controling micoorganisms.
4. What are various physical methods of sterilization? What are its advantages and disadvantages?
5. Write an essay on chemotherapy and antibiotics.

6. **What is asepsis? Differentiate between medical and surgical asepsis?**
7. **Write Short Notes:**
   - Medical and Surgical Asepsis
   - Pasteurization
   - Autoclave
   - Chemical Sterilization
   - Sterilization
   - Radiation Sterilization
   - Chemotherapy
   - Antibiotics
   - Principles of Surgical Asepsiss
   - Cross infection
   - Technique of handwashing
   - Surgical team
   - Personal Hygiene
   - Asepsis Dry heat and moist heat

Chapter

14

Biosafety and Waste Management

■ BIOSAFETY

Biosafety means efforts done by us to ensure safety while using, transporting, transferring, releasing and disposing parts or whole of organisms.

Many countries proposed strict laws and regulations to avoid any harm that happen due to lack of biosafety. However, even few other countries lack biosafety awareness and thus they create problems to the as well as to the environment.

■ NEED FOR BIOSAFETY

Coming in contact with human blood or blood products or with certain harmful chemicals used in laboratories is potentially dangerous (technically called hazardous). Biosafety involves taking precautions to protect you and co-workers against infection, injury or even poisoning.

Most policy and regulatory activities under Biosafety are local limited to Nations. However, International agreements are found essential to make all Nations equal and to standardize the rules of Biosafety throughout the earth. Certain Organizations deal with different rule sets of Biosafety. For instance, FAO deals with risks associated with environment and food under Biosafety. The organization also helps in providing Sanitary and Phytosanitary (meaning sanitation through plants) measures (SPS). It develops methods for analysing risks in food and agriculture industry, fisheries and forestry as well.

■ TERMS USED IN BIOSAFETY

Stability: The ability of chemical to stay strong without getting decomposed.

Incompatibility: Certain chemicals should not be mixed or even stored together which may create dangerous consequences.

Hazardous Decomposition Products: Harmful chemical products formed when chemicals decomposes of burns.

Hazardous Polymerization: Accumulation of more likely harmful substances is called hazardous polymerization. This enhances the severity of consequences. It causes more heat to be released which might explode the containers.

Accessibility: Ensured sites are secure to limit unauthorised or unintentional access.

Clear Access: if the waste collection point is inside the work area, access to the area shall be kept clean. A dedicated chemical waste storage area should be considered.

Signage: Signage should be erected advising the location of collection point.

Conditions: Collection points and storage areas shall be cool, dry and free from contamination.

Cleaning: Floors shall be smooth and impervious for easy cleaning. A water supply shall be in close proximity for cleaning purposes.

Ventilation: Natural or mechanical ventilation shall be provided to prevent build-up of fumes and vapours.

Location: Shall be sited away from food preparation, smoking or storage areas.

Drainage: Drainage systems shall not allow run-off from spills, etc. to enter storm-water drains.

Security: Collection points must be secured at all time when not in use.

Arrangement shall be established to provide waste contractors with accessibility for collection of waste.

■ SPILL, LEAK AND DISPOSAL PROCEDURES

When accidental spills, leaks or disposal of harmful chemicals happen while you work in laboratory, there are certain procedures which need to be followed. These procedures include appropriate waste disposal methods required for safety and environmental protection.

Eye protection: Recommendations are dependent upon the irritancy, corrosivity and special handling procedures.

Skin protection: describes the particular types of protective garments and appropriate glove materials to provide personnel protection

Respiratory protection: appropriate respirators for conditions exceeding the recommended occupational exposure limits.

■ BIOSAFETY CABINETS AND OTHER SAFETY EQUIPMENTS (FIGURES 14.1 AND 14.2)

Biological Safety Cabinets (BSC) prevents the contamination of harmful microorganisms in air while working with highly infectious materials inside the Laminar flow chamber. Among various types of classes available for Biological Safety Cabinets, only Class II BSC is mostly preferred. The followings are instruments used for providing additional protection through Biosafety.

Chemical Fume Hoods: Protect the environment from vapours and gases

Biological Safety Cabinets: Protect the environment from small particles

Clean Benches: For doing work comfortably with maximum sterility.

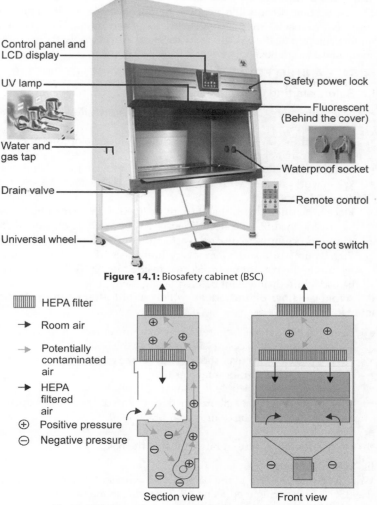

Figure 14.1: Biosafety cabinet (BSC)

Figure 14.2: Internal view of biological safety cabinet (BSC)

■ BIOSAFETY CABINET ALARMS

Try not to work with Biosafety Cabinets connected to Alarming System. This Alarming system is necessary for those laboratories where biosafety is not practised absolutely. When alarm rings, it says that there are certain spills, leakages or even contamination happened. Make sure that you get out of the laboratory to protect yourself from infections.

■ OTHER SAFETY EQUIPMENTS

The use of some devices like blenders, homogenizers, sonicators produce aerosols. "Aerosols" means small particles mixed in air. These aerosols might contaminate the BSC. To reduce exposure to aerosols, these devices should be used in BSC only when it is really necessary.

■ SAFE AND EFFECTIVE USE OF THE BIOSAFETY CABINET (BSC)

I. Before starting the work in laboratory:

- Check Biosafety Cabinet Alarms, pressure gauges, flow indicators for any changes.
- Switch off the UV-light otherwise, you might get skin cancer as UV-light is a carcinogen.
- Switch on the Biosafety Cabinet and allow it to run for 3-5 minutes.
- Wipe work surface with an appropriate disinfectant. Mostly 90% alcohol is preferred.
- Place a pan filled with disinfectant or lined with a small biohazard bag inside the BSC to collect discards. Avoid reaching outside of BSC during procedures to discard waste in floor containers.
- Plan your work and place everything needed for the procedure including the pan for your discards inside the BSC. Wipe all items to be used with disinfectant before placing them in BSC.

II. Avoid air flow disturbances which might affect the protection level in BSC:

- Keep the BSC free of clutter like extra unwanted equipments and supplies. Keep all necessary items only in the BSC.
- Do not place objects over the front air intake grille.
- Do not block the rear air intake grille.
- Do not allow more people to be near BSC when it is in use.
- Always check whether laboratory door is closed. Try to avoid opening and closing door if the door is near BSC.
- Work slowly.
- Do not operate a Bunsen Burner inside the BSC.

III. While working:

Work as far as possible to the back of BSC workspace as possible. Dont use BSC for preparing media and all. Try to finish majority of your steps outside BSC.

Separate contaminated and clean items. Work from "Clean to dirty".
Clean up all spills in the cabinet immediately then and there when it happens. Allow cabinet to run for 3–5 minutes before resuming work when there is any spill.

IV. After completing the work:

Wipe down all items with an appropriate disinfectant before removing. Remove all materials and wipe the interior surfaces with the same.
Check for the decontaminates in regular intervals under work grilles.

■ GENERAL LABORATORY SAFETY (FIGURE: 14.3)

- Laboratory employees must notify immediately to the laboratory manager or PI in case of an accident, injury, illness, or overt exposure associated with laboratory activities.
- No eating, drinking, smoking, handling contact lenses or applying cosmetics in the laboratory at any time.
- No animals or minors (persons under the age of 18), or Immuno-compromised persons will be allowed to enter the laboratory at any time.
- Food, medications or cosmetics should not be brought into the laboratory for storage or later use. Food is stored outside in areas designated specifically for that purpose.
- No open-toed shoes or sandals are allowed in the laboratory.
- Personal Protective Equipments (PPE) includes gloves, lab coat and eye protection.
- All skin defects such as cuts, abrasions, ulcers, areas of dermatitis, etc. should be covered with an air tight and water proof bandage.
- Pipetting out solutions by mouth is prohibited; mechanical pipetting devices are to be used at all times.
- All procedures are to be performed carefully to minimize the creation of splashes or aerosols.
- Follow all manufacturer's instructions and Standard Operating Procedures (SOPs) when using any of the laboratory equipment.
- Wash hands: After removing gloves and before leaving the laboratory.
- Razor blades, scalpels, and hypodermic needles ("sharps") should be discarded into the "sharps" container in the biosafety cabinet. Needles should not be recapped.
- Work surfaces will be decontaminated as needed with. Follow manufacturer instructions for contact time.
- All cultures, stocks and other regulated wastes are decontaminated by autoclaving before disposal. Liquids (non-organic) can be decontaminated with bleach, bringing the solution to 10% bleach, and discarded in the sink. No other chemicals can be discarded in the sink.

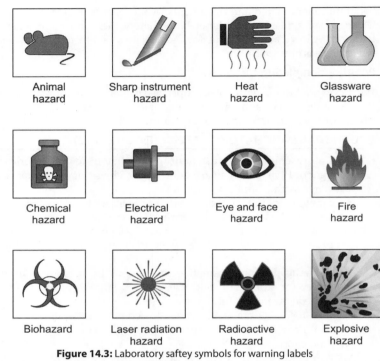

Figure 14.3: Laboratory saftey symbols for warning labels

◼ WASTE DISPOSAL

Waste is anything that is not required for us and must be discarded. Decontamination of wastes and their ultimate disposal are closely interrelated. Most glassware, instruments and laboratory clothing will be reused or recycled. The overriding principle is that all infectious materials should be decontaminated (meaning: removed with harmful microorganisms or organisms or harmful chemicals), autoclaved (meaning: heated to high temperature about 121°C for 15 minutes at 15lbs) or incinerated (meaning: burnt in high temperature to ash) within the laboratory. The principal question that hints our mind before discharge of any objects or materials by laboratory workers who deal with highly infectious microorganisms or animal tissues:

- Have the objects or materials been effectively decontaminated or disinfected by an approved procedure?
- If not, have they been packaged in an approved manner for immediate on-site incineration or transfer to another facility with incineration capacity?

- Does the disposal of the decontaminated objects or materials involve any additional potential hazards, biological or otherwise, to those who carry out the immediate disposal procedures or who might come into contact with discarded items outside the facility?

PROPER DISPOSAL OF SHARPS AND WASTES

- Take precautions to avoid needle stick injury which can be caused due to several reasons including lack of focus, inexperience, lack of concern for others, improper disposal of sharps, etc.
- Always drop used sharps in special containers.
- Do not break, bend, re-sheath or reuse lancets, syringes or needles.
- Do not shake sharps containers to create space.
- Never place needles or sharps in Office waste containers.
- Sharps containers must be placed near workspace closed when not in use. Usually, these sharps containers should be sealed three quarters to avoid injuries.

POLICY FOR HANDLING SHARPS

- User is responsible for disposal of sharps.
- Must dispose of sharps after each test.
- Must place sharps in sharps boxes.
- Do not drop sharps on the floor or in the Office waste bin.
- Place sharps container near your workspace.
- Seal and remove when box is three quarters full.
- Incinerate all waste.

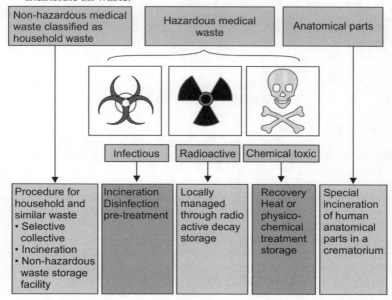

Handling Chemicals

Chemicals are sometimes ignitable, corrosive, reactive or toxic. Therefore, they should be handled properly. In case there is any spill of chemicals then do the following: Paper towels are to be applied to absorb the spill, and then paper towels are soaked with any of the disinfectants. For spills outside the bio-safety hood, alert others in the area. Use N95 mask if there is a possibility of harmful aerosols. All aspects of the emergency SOPs are followed without exception.

■ DISINFECTION

- Always disinfectants are used to kill germs and pathogens to keep the work surface clean.
- Disinfection prevents cross contamination and reduces risk of infection

■ HAZARDOUS CHEMICAL WASTES

Hazardous chemical wastes may be in liquid, solid or gaseous form and include:

- Laboratory chemical waste
- Chemically contaminated consumables such as broken laboratory equipment, heavily contaminated personal protective environment (PPE) and bench covers
- Other by-products resulting from the use of hazardous chemicals
- Commercial or industrial waste or construction and demolition waste contaminated with or is a substance.

■ DECONTAMINATION

Steam autoclaving can be used for waste decontamination. Simply all the materials are to be placed and disposed in the containers. These are then placed in autoclave. There are certain commercially available plastic bags which can be used for carrying all the above mentioned materials for autoclaving. This method kills microorganisms, however not spores. Some laboratories choose incineration method (burning things to ash) for waste disposal.

There are some materials and equipments which cannot be autoclaved. For these materials and equipments you can use chemical disinfectants for removing harmful organisms or harmful chemicals. Depending on the resistance of harmful organisms contained in wastes the disinfectant can be choosen. Using chemical disinfectants can easily kill vegetative bacteria, fungi and enveloped viruses while Mycobacteria and non-enveloped viruses are killed slowly. Other organisms like bacterial spores and protozoan cysts cannot be killed by disinfectants.

Gamma irradiation is another method of killing harmful organisms and also decontaminating heat sensitive materials. Depending on the density of waste materials and strength of gamma irradiation source, the efficiency of treatment can be determined.

Finally, incineration has traditionally been the chosen method for destroying anatomical biomedical waste and animal carcasses. In most cases, wastes to be incinerated have to be packaged and transported off-site in accordance with provincial or territorial legislation. Steam autoclaving of materials should be done initially, only then followed by incineration.

THE HANDLING AND DISPOSAL OF CONTAMINATED MATERIALS AND WASTES

There should be identification and separation system for infectious materials and their containers. Since there are no stringent national regulations; international regulations best practices must be followed. Categories should include:

- non-contaminated (non-infectious) waste that can be reused or recycled or disposed of as general, "household" waste.
- contaminated (infectious) "sharps" – hypodermic needles, scalpels, knives and broken glass; should always be collected in puncture-proof containers fitted with covers and treated as infectious.
- contaminated material for decontamination by autoclaving and thereafter washing and reuse or recycling.
- contaminated material for autoclaving and disposal.
- contaminated material for direct incineration.

SHARPS

After use, hypodermic needles should not be recapped, clipped removed from disposable syringes. The complete assembly should be placed in a sharps disposal container. Disposable syringes, used alone or with needles, should be placed in sharps disposal containers and incinerated with prior autoclaving if required. Sharps disposal containers must be puncture-proof-resistant and must not be filled to capacity. When they are three-quarters full they should be placed in "infectious waste" containers and incinerated with prior autoclaving. Sharps disposal containers must not be discarded in landfills.

CONTAMINATED (POTENTIALLY INFECTIOUS) MATERIALS FOR AUTOCLAVING AND REUSE

No pre-cleaning should be attempted if any contaminated or potentially infectious materials are to be autoclaved and reused. Any necessary cleaning or repair must be done only after autoclaving or disinfection.

CONTAMINATED MATERIALS FOR DISPOSAL

Apart from sharps, all contaminated materials should be autoclaved in leak proof containers, example autoclavable, colour-coded plastic bags, before disposal. After autoclaving, the material may be placed in transfer containers for transport to the incinerator. If possible, materials deriving from healthcare activities should not be discarded in landfills even after decontamination.

▌ PROCESS FOR HAZARDOUS CHEMICALS WASTE MANAGEMENT (TABLE 14.1)

Waste Characterization

- Dangerous by-products may result when mixing incompatible waste categories.
- To ensure safe storage, handling and disposal of hazardous chemical waste, work area managers shall ensure producing chemical waste mixtures record ingredient information and properties of the waste (e.g. corrosive, flammable or other specific hazards).
- This information should be followed by workers, waste contractors and others who likely to work with any of the hazardous chemical wastes.

Waste Segregation

- Hazardous chemical waste shall be segregated according to hazard class and waste category.
- Mixed hazard classes include chemical wastes of differing hazard classes which shall not be mixed. For instance, concentrated acids or alkalis shall not be mixed with other chemicals.
- Mixed waste categories – where the chemical waste may belong to more than one waste category the following guide shall be used:
  - Radioactive and chemical waste – treat as radioactive waste in the first instance.
  - Clinical and chemical waste – if grossly contaminated with biological material treat as clinical in the first instance.

On-site Collection, Transport and Storage

- Chemical waste, and in particular flammable or combustible liquid waste, shall not be allowed to accumulate and regular collections shall be established.
- When establishing regular waste collections consideration shall be given to
  - Appropriateness of waste receptacles and containers
  - Frequency of collection
  - Collection points and storage sitting
  - Container management
  - Containment of spills and leaks
  - On-site transport
  - Accessibility of SDS

- Where practicable, transportation shall be scheduled for non-peak traffic times and consideration given to the following:
  - Route and method of transport
  - Use trolleys or carts that are easy to load, unload and clean
  - Transport equipment shall be free of sharp edges or protrusions that may puncture container
  - Equipment shall regularly be cleaned to remove any chemical residues and reduce exposure risks
  - Containment of smaller drums / bottles within plastic tubs (for fume and spill containment)
  - Use of original packaging or specific packaging to limit damage during transport (e.g. Glass Winchesters used in laboratories).

Container Management

Containers utilised as part of waste management shall:
- be maintained in good condition at all times
- be securely closed at all times unless adding or removing waste
- only be filled to three quarters full to allow for contraction or expansion of the contents
- be appropriate for the type of waste to be collected
- Khall, if practicable, be legibly labelled with the following:
  - Product identifier
  - Name, Address and Telephone number of the manufacturer or importer
  - Hazard classification (e.g. oxidising liquid)
  - A hazard pictogram and hazard statement consistent with the classification of the chemical.
  - Glass containers shall be packaged to minimise risk of breakage.

Empty Containers

- Empty waste containers that cannot safely be decontaminated shall be treated as chemical waste and stored at a secured collection point.
- Labels shall be left on containers which are unable to be properly decontaminated.
- Empty gas cylinders shall be returned to the vendor for reuse or disposal.
- Option for dealing with empty containers are:
  - Option 1 – return to the vendor for re-use or disposal
  - Option 2 – disposal to general or recycling waste.

If option 2 is adopted, the container shall be completely empty and triple rinsed with water to remove residual material and vapours. The rinse water used for cleaning may need to be contained for treatment or packaged as chemical waste for collection and disposal.

Table 14.1: Different types of wastes including hazardous wastes

Term	Definition / Explanation / Details	Term	Definition / Explanation / Details
Clinical Waste	Waste that has the potential to cause disease, including for example animal waste, discarded sharps, human tissue waste, laboratory waste, etc. Note: Clinical waste does not include waste from laboratories that do not conduct testing of blood, body fluids or tissues from humans or animals	Hazardous chemical	Means 'a substance, mixture or article that satisfied the criteria for a hazard class in the Globally Harmonised System (GHS)' and may include radioactive and waste chemicals or other material contaminated with hazardous chemicals.
Cytotoxic waste	Material that is, or may be, contaminated by a cytotoxic medication	Hazardous chemical waste	Waste generated from the use of hazardous chemicals in workplace procedures. This includes procedures undertaken in laboratories, workshops, oral health and clinical services and other functional areas.
Dangerous Goods	Goods are dangerous goods if they are defined under the Australian Dangerous Goods (ADG) Code as dangerous goods; or goods too dangerous to be transported.	Sharps	Objects or devices having sharp points or protuberances or cutting edges, capable of cutting or piercing the skin. Includes hypodermic, intravenous or other medical needles, Pasteur pipettes, scalpel blades, lancets, scissors, glass slides, broken glass such as vials, bottles and laboratory glass.

Cont...

Cont...

Term	Definition / Explanation / Details	Term	Definition / Explanation / Details
Environmental harm	Any adverse effect, or potential adverse effect (whether temporary or permanent and of whatever magnitude, duration or frequency) on an environmental value, and includes environmental nuisance. Note: Material and serious environmental harm denote varying degrees of environmental harm.	Related waste	Waste that constitutes, or is contaminated with, chemicals, cytotoxic drugs, human body parts, pharmaceutical products or radioactive substances.
General Waste	Waste other than regulated waste	Regulated waste	Means waste that is or contains a substance, or residues of a substance
Industrial waste	Is interceptor waste or waste other than commercial waste; domestic cleanup and domestic waste; green waste; recyclable interceptor waste; recyclable waste; waste discharged to sewer.	Laboratory waste	A specimen or culture discarded in the course of dental, medical or veterinary practice or research, including material that is, or has been contaminated by, genetically manipulated material or imported biological material.

■ POSSIBLE QUESTIONS

1. Define biosafety and explain its needs.
2. Why mouth pipetting is strictly prohibited?
3. Using disinfectants to clean your work surface is highly helpful to keep you healthy. Justify the statement.
4. What is hazardous waste? In which form, you can see hazardous waste?
5. Mention the steps involved in the process of hazardous waste management.
6. Enumerate different types of waste and its management.

7. **Write Short Notes:**
   - Biosafety
   - Biological safety cabinet (BSC)
   - General laboratory safety
   - Hospital waste disposal
   - Types of medical waste
   - Disinfection
   - Decontamination
   - Container Management

Chapter

15

Introduction to Laboratory Techniques

■ INTRODUCTION

Microorganisms are present everywhere in nature. They are seen in soil, air, water, food, sewage and on body surfaces. The main aim of every microbiologists is to separate these mixtures of different microorganism populations into individual group of species for their studies. A culture containing only a single species of microorganism is referred to as pure culture. For isolation and studies on microorganisms as pure culture, the microbiologists need various basic laboratory equipments and techniques as shown in the following table:

Table 15.1: Different laboratory apparatus and techniques used in microbiology laboratory

Laboratory Apparatus	Techniques Used
Media	For isolation of Pure cultures:
Autoclave	Streak plate
Bunsen burner	Pour plate – loop dilution
Culture tubes	Spread plate
Petri dishes	
Pipettes	Staining methods:
Water baths	Simple staining – negative staining
Incubators	Differential staining – Gram staining and Acid fast staining
Refrigerators	
Wood Chamber	
Inoculation tube	
Culture flasks	
Wire loops and needles	

■ APPARATUS IN MICROBIOLOGY LABORATORY

Media (Figures 15.1 (A to E))

- Growing bacteria under artificial conditions in the laboratory is called as culturing.
- To culture bacteria we provide them nutrients through media called as growth media or culture media.
- There are various reasons why we have to culture bacteria in the laboratory on artificial culture media.
- One of the most important reasons being its utility in diagnosing infectious diseases.

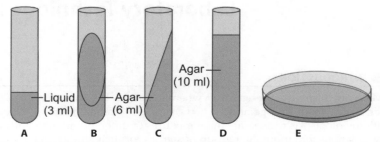

Figures 15.1 (A to E): Different forms of Media, (A) Broth medium, (B) Agar slant – front view (C) Agar slant – side view (D) Agar deep tube and (E) Agar plate or petridish

Culture Tubes and Petri Dishes

- Glass test tubes and glass based or even plastic based Petri dishes are widely used for cultivating microorganisms.
- Glass tubes are found to be suitable for both solid and liquid forms of nutrient medium while Petri dishes are suitable only for solid medium.
- There are different closures available to maintain sterility in these medium tubes and Petri dishes.
- Schroeder and von Dusch was the first person to develop a very good closure type called cotton plug.
- Cotton plug is used to cover the test tube in avoiding contamination. Microorganisms grown in the test tube also need oxygen. Cotton plug allows Oxygen to pass through and so, microorganism grows better.
- However, preparing sterile cotton plugs is difficult which should be done inside the laminar hood.
- Commercially available sleeve-like caps are helpful in replacing cotton plugs.
- Most laboratories prefer sleeve-like caps than cotton plugs.
- Petri dish is the apparatus which has two parts. One is the top portion which is bigger in size and the other is the bottom portion which is smaller in size.

- As both parts are not matching perfectly, there is a gap between these two parts when closed. Through this gap the air can enter the Petri dish and microorganism can grow better.

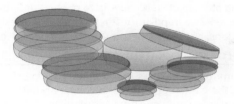

Figure 15.2: Petri dishes

Transfer Instruments

- Microorganisms must be transferred from one vessel to another for maintenance and study.
- Such a transfer is called as **subculturing** and must be carried out under sterile conditions to prevent possible combination.
- Wire loops and needles are made from inert metals such as Nichrome or Platinum and are inserted into metal shafts that serve as handles.
- They are extremely durable instruments and are easily sterilized by incineration in the blue (hottest) portion of the Bunsen burner flame.
- A pipette is another instrument used for sterile transfers.
- Pipettes are similar in function to straws; that is, they draw up liquids. They are made up of glass or plastic drawn out to a tip at one end and with a mouthpiece forming the other end.

Cultivation Chambers

- The most important requirement for the cultivation of microorganisms is that they can be grown at their optimum temperature. An incubator is used to maintain optimum temperature during the necessary growth period.
- Most incubators use dry heat. Moisture is supplied by placing a beaker of water in the incubator during the growth period. A moist environment retards dehydration of the medium and thereby avoids spurious experimental results.
- A heat controlled shaking water bath is another piece of apparatus used to cultivate microorganisms. Its advantage is that it provides a rapid and uniform transfer of heat to the culture vessel and its agitation provides increased aeration, resulting in acceleration of growth. The single disadvantage of this instrument is that it can be used only for cultivation of organisms in a broth medium.

Refrigerator

- A refrigerator is used for a wide variety of purposes such as maintenance and storage of stock cultures between subculturing periods and storage of sterile media to prevent dehydration.
- It is also used as a repository for thermolabile (destroyed by high heat) solutions, antibiotics, serums and biochemical reagents.

■ ISOLATION OF MICROORGANISMS

In nature, at any place, various microorganisms co-exist as a group. In the laboratory, these microorganisms can be separated into pure cultures. These cultures contain only one type of organism and are suitable for the study of their cultural, morphological and biochemical properties.

The followings are techniques that can be used to accomplish this necessary dilution:

Streak Plate Method

The streak plate method is a rapid qualitative isolation method. It is essentially a dilution technique that involves spreading a loopful of culture over the surface of an agar plate. Although many types of procedures are performed, the four-way or quadrant, streak is explained as follows:

(Ensure to follow all these steps inside the Laminar Air Flow Hood)

- Take the inoculation loop. Hold it upright. Show the loop in the flame of Bunsen burner until it turns red hot. Allow it to cool by keeping it in your right hand for few seconds (10-20 preferably).
- Hold the culture tube in your left hand. Using smaller finger and palm of your right hand open the cotton plug from the culture tube.
- Insert the cooled loop into the culture tube to collect the sample.
- Swipe the loop onto the surface of culture tube. Now you will get a loopful of culture.
- Then, close the culture tube with cotton plug using the same smaller finger and palm.
- Then, take Petri dish containing only Media on your left hand and open it slowly.
- Now gently place the loopful of culture at one end of the media. 'A' as shown in the following figure (Figure 15.3).
- Spread the culture perpendicularly like lines in two directions using the same loop continuously.
- Repeat "step a" to sterilize inoculation loop.
- From the end of lines in A, you have to spread the culture again perpendicularly like lines in two directions using the same loop continuously. This is referred to as "B".
- Repeat "step a" to sterilize inoculation loop.

- From the end of lines in B, you have to spread the culture again perpendicularly like lines in two directions using the same loop continuously. This is referred to as "C".
- Repeat "step a" to sterilize inoculation loop.
- From the end of lines in C, you have to spread the culture again perpendicularly like lines in two directions using the same loop continuously. This is referred to as "D".
- Repeat "step a" to sterilize inoculation loop.
- From the end of lines in D, you have to spread the culture again perpendicularly like lines in two directions using the same loop continuously. This is referred to as "E".
- Repeat "step a" to sterilize inoculation loop. Keep the inoculation loop aside.
- Now, individual colonies of microorganisms are separated in E.

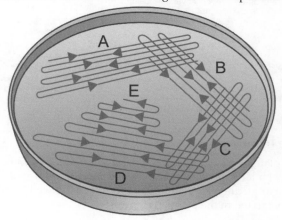

Figure 15.3: Streak plate method for isolation of pure culture

Spread Plate Technique

The spread-plate technique requires that a previously diluted mixture of microorganisms be used. During inoculation, the cells are spread over the surface of a solid agar medium with a sterile, L-shaped bent rod while the Petri dish is spun on a "Lazy-Susan" turntable. The step by step procedure for this technique includes:
(Make sure you do all these steps inside the Laminar Air Flow Hood)
- Take the sterile beaker containing nutrient broth with single colony of microorganism on your left hand.
- Using smaller finger and palm of your right hand open the cotton plug from the sterile beaker.
- Insert the sterile pipette into the nutrient broth containing beaker

to pipette out the sample culture. (You should not pipette out the sample culture by mouth. Using pointing finger of your right hand try pipetting out sample culture)

▪ Then using smaller finger and palm of your right hand close the cotton plug over the sterile beaker.

▪ Take sterile Petri dish containing agar media and pour the sample culture over the agar surface.

▪ Using sterile glass spreader spread the culture evenly all over the Petri plate by rotating the spreader at 360°.

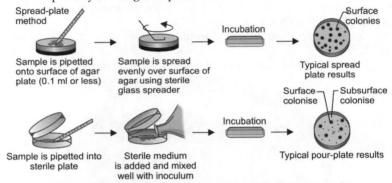

Figure 15.4: Spread plate and pour plate method of isolating pure culture

Pour Plate Technique

The pour plate technique requires a serial dilution of the mixed culture by means of a loop or pipette. The diluted inoculums are then added to a molten agar medium in a Petri dish, mixed and allowed to solidify. It is well demonstrated in the picture (Figure 15.4).

Pipette Transfer

The procedure for carrying out pipette transfer includes the following:

▪ Tilt a can of pipettes so that the tops of the pipettes are at the top of can.

▪ Set the can on the laboratory bench so that the top of the can extends off the edge of bench.

▪ Remove the lid from the can and set the lid on countertop.

▪ Without removing it from the can, pick up a pipette with your non-dominant hand. Use your dominant hand to place a pipette aid on the pipette.

▪ Slide the pipette from the can, lifting it to avoid dragging the bottom of the pipette across the contaminated surfaces of other pipettes.

▪ Use the little finger of the hand holding the pipette to remove the lid from the container containing your sample.

- Touch the tip of pipette to the side of container.
- Measure the sample into the container.
- Place the pipette into a discard container and remove the pipette aid.

■ PURE CULTURE TECHNIQUES

After getting pure culture from any of the three methods as seen above, the culture needs to be sub-cultured by transferring them into a new medium. This would ensure continuous growth and division of microorganisms. Also, you can have the live culture. Microorganisms are transferred from one medium to another by subculturing. These techniques are very basic for all microbiology experiments which include preparation of stock cultures and their maintenance.

Microorganisms are always present in the air and on laboratory surfaces, benches and equipment. They can serve as a source of external contamination and thus interfere with experimental results unless proper techniques are used during subculturing. It includes the following:

- Sterilize the inoculation loop by holding it in the flame of Bunsen burner until it turns red hot. This is the very basic step used more frequently. While doing this, caution must be taken in order to sterilize the inoculation loop. Then, the inoculation loop should be placed in your hand for 10-20 seconds to cool. The stock culture tube and the tube to be inoculated need to be placed in the same hand. It would look like V in hand which represents two test tubes: one with culture tube and another tube to be inoculated.
- Using the little finger to grasp the first cap tightly for uncapping and with the next finger try to remove the cap of another tube. Insert the sterile inoculation loop into the cultured tube to collect the sample and then insert the same loop into the test tube which contains only media. Then, close the caps one by one.
- After completing this step, again sterilize the inoculation loop by holding it in the flame of Bunsen burner. This is to kill any organisms that are left in the loop.

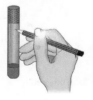

A. With a wax pencil label the medium to be inoculated | **B.** Shake the primary culture tube to suspend the bacteria | **C.** Place both tubes in the palm of one hand to fom A V

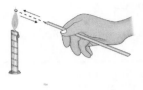

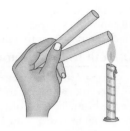

D. Place both tubes in the palm of one hand to fom A V

E. Remove the caps from the tubes and flame the necks of the tubes

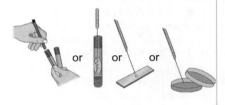

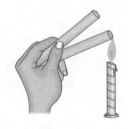

F. Cool the loop or needle and pick up bacteria	Streak the surface of a slant	Place the bacteria on slide	Streak the bacteria on plate

G. Remove the necks of the tubes

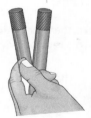

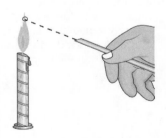

H. Flecap the tubes

I. Remove the loop or needle

Figures 15.5 (A to I): Method of subculturing

■ CULTURE MEDIA

Need for culture media

It is usually essential to obtain a culture by growing the organism in an artificial medium. If more than one species or type of organism is present, each requires to be separated carefully or isolated as pure culture. Several organisms need the determination of antibiotic sensitivity pattern for optimal antibiotic selection.

Types of Culture Media

Table 15.2: Description of raw materials used in culture media with its nutritional value

Raw Material	Characteristic	Nutritional Value
Beef extract	An aqueous extract of lean beef tissue concentrated to a paste	Contains the water-soluble substances of animal tissue, which include carbohydrates, organic nitrogen compounds, water-soluble vitamins and salts
Peptone	The product resulting from the digestion of proteinaceous materials example, meat, casein and gelatin; digestion of the protein material is accomplished with acids or enzymes; many different peptones (depending upon the protein used and the method of digestion) are available for use in bacteriological media; peptones differ in their ability to support growth of bacteria.	Principal source of organic nitrogen; may also contain some vitamins and sometimes carbohydrates, depending upon the kind of proteinaceous material digested.
Agar	A complex carbohydrate obtained from certain marine algae; processed to remove extraneous substances	Used as a solidification agent for media; agar, dissolved in aqueous solutions, gels when the temperature is reduced below 45°C; agar not considered a source of nutrient to the bacteria

Cont...

Cont...

Raw Material	Characteristic	Nutritional Value
Yeast extract	An aqueous extract of yeast cells, commercially available as a powder	A very rich source of the B vitamins; also contains organic nitrogen and carbon compounds.

Table 15.3: Composition of nutrient broth and nutrient agar

Nutrient Broth	Beef extract – 3 g Peptone – 5 g Water – 1000 ml
Nutrient Agar	Beef extract – 3 g Peptone – 5 g Agar – 15 g Water – 1000 ml

Table 15.4: Types of culture media

Based on their consistency	Solid medium Liquid medium Semi solid medium
Based on the constituents or ingredients	Simple medium Complex medium Synthetic or defined medium Special medium (includes enriched media, enrichment media, selective media, indicator media, differential media, transport media)
Based on Oxygen requirement	Aerobic media Anaerobic media

Based on their consistency

Solid media- Solid media has agar in concentration of 1.5 to 2%. Example: Nutrient Agar.

Liquid Media: Liquid media does not have agar. Example: Nutrient Broth.

Semisolid Media: Semisolid media has agar in concentration less than 0.5%. The media looks very soft like jelly. Example: Fluid thioglycollate media.

Based on the constituents or ingredients

Basal Media/ Simple Media– Such are basically simple media that supports non-fastidious bacteria. Peptone water, nutrient broth and nutrient agar are considered as basal media. These media are generally used for the primary isolation of microorganisms. Examples: Peptone Water, nutrient broth, nutrient agar, etc.

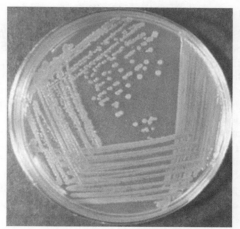

Figure 15.6: Bacteria grown on simple media (Nutrient Agar)

Synthetic or chemically defined media– A chemically defined medium is one prepared from purified ingredients and therefore whose exact composition is known. Example- Minimal media for *Bacillus megaterium*.

Complex media– Non-synthetic medium contains at least one component that is neither purified nor completely known. Often these are partially digested proteins from various organism sources. Example- Nutrient Broth

Enriched Media (Added Growth Factors) Figure: 15.7– When basal media contains special ingredients like blood, serum, egg yolk, etc, then the medium is considered as enriched media. Example: Chocolate agar, blood agar, etc.

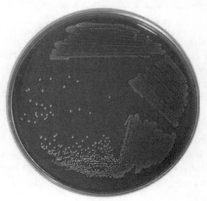

Figure 15.7: Enriched media (Blood Agar)

Selective and enrichment media

These are designed to inhibit unwanted commensal or contaminating bacteria and help to recover pathogen from a mixture of bacteria. While selective media are agar based and enrichment media are liquid in consistency. Both these media serve the same purpose. Any agar media can be made selective by addition of certain inhibitory agents that don't affect the pathogen. Various approaches to make a medium selective include addition of antibiotics, dyes, chemicals, alteration of pH or a combination of these.

Selective media (Figure 15.8): Selective medium is designed to suppress the growth of some microorganisms while allowing the growth of others (i.e., they select for certain microbes). Solid medium is employed with selective medium so that individual colonies may be isolated. Examples of selective media include: Thayer Martin Agar used to recover *N.gonorrhoeae* contains Vancomycin, Colistin and Nystatin.

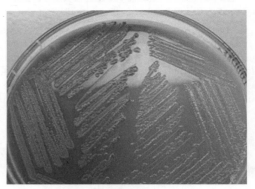

Figure 15.8: Thayer Martin Agar

Enrichment Media: Enrichment medium is used to increase the relative concentration of certain microorganisms in the culture prior to plating on solid selective medium. Unlike selective media, enrichment culture is typically used as broth medium. Enrichment media are liquid media that also serves to inhibit commensals in the clinical specimen. Example, Selenite F broth, Tetrathionate broth and Alkaline peptone water are used to recover pathogens from fecal specimens.

Differential Media: Special type of media used for differentiating two varieties of bacteria or other microorganisms is called Differential media. Differentiation of two bacterial colonies can be identified through various methods including dye absorption, metabolism, etc. Example – MacConkey Agar.

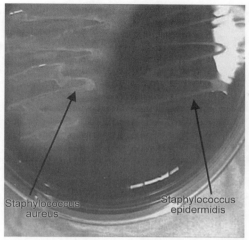

Figure 15.9: Differential medium – MacConkey Agar

Transport Media: Clinical specimens must be transported to the laboratory immediately after collection to prevent overgrowth of contaminating organisms or commensals. This can be achieved by using transport media. Transport media should fulfil the following criteria:

- Temporary storage of specimens being transported to the laboratory for cultivation.
- Maintain the viability of all organisms in the specimen without altering their concentration.
- Contain only buffers and salts.
- Lack of carbon, nitrogen and organic growth factors so as to prevent microbial multiplication.
- Transport media used in the isolation of anaerobes much be free of molecular Oxygen.

Examples: Cary Blair Media for *Campylobacter*

Assay media: These media are used for the assay of Vitamins, Amino acids and antibiotics, e.g. Antibiotic assay media are used for determining antibiotic potency by the microbiological assay technique.

Other types of Media include Media for Enumeration of Bacteria, Media for characterization of Bacteria, Maintenance media etc.

Based on the oxygen requirement

Aerobic media- Media which contains oxygen are called Aerobic media. All the above seen media fall under this group.

Anaerobic media (Figure: 15.10)- Anaerobic bacteria need special media for growth because they need low Oxygen content, reduced oxidation – reduction potential and extra nutrients. Media for anaerobes may have to be supplemented with nutrients like hemin and vitamin K. Such media may also have to be reduced by physical or chemical means.

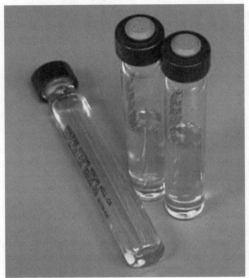

Figure 15.10: Anaerobic media

■ INOCULATION OF CULTURE MEDIA

For all microbiological experiments, we need good techniques for separating our desired sample from culture media. This is very important to study the characteristics of sample organism. Several modified techniques are available depending on the needs of the microbiologists. All commercially available culture media should be checked whether they are pure or contaminated along with the details of their expiry date. This is also very important as contaminated culture media might facilitate the growth of unwanted organism when sample organisms are grown. After expiry date when the culture media is used that might affect the growth of the sample organisms. It is very easy to identify the plates which exceed expiry date or even contaminated plates as the media might become turbid.

Inoculation loops can be sterilized by holding the loop end shown in the flame of Bunsen burner until the loop turns red hot. Then the inoculation loop is kept on the rack for cooling before being used. If the inoculation loop in red hot is used, then the microorganisms would die in hotness. For every plate different disposable inoculation loops can be used. When transfer of colonies between test tubes happen, every time the loop should be sterilized by showing it to the flame of Bunsen burner.

Aseptic Transfer

Specific transfer methods

There are two basic stages in transfers: 1) obtaining the sample to be transferred and 2) transferring to the sterile culture medium. These may be combined in various ways. The following descriptions are organized to reflect that flexibility.

- Materials are neatly positioned and not in the way. To prevent spills, culture tubes are stored upright in a test tube rack. They are never laid on the table. The microbiologist is relaxed and ready for work. He should hold the loop like a pencil, not gripping it like a dagger.
- Incineration of an inoculating loop's wire is done by passing it through the tip of the flame's inner cone. Begin at the wire's base and continue to the end making sure that all parts are heated to a uniform orange color: Allow the wire to cool before touching it or placing it on/in a culture. The former will burn and latter will cause aerosols of microorganisms.
- Remove the tube's cap with your little finger by pulling the tube away with the other hand; the loop hand is kept still. The cap should be hold with little finger during the transfer. When replacing the cap, always move the tube back to the cap in order to keep your loop hand still. The replaced cap doesn't need to be on firmly yet – just enough to cover the tube.
- The open tube should be hold on an angle to minimize the chance that airborne microbes will drop into it. The tube's mouth will quickly be passed through the flame a couple of times. The tube's cap being held in the loop hand is to be noticed.

■ TRANSFERS USING AN INOCULATING LOOP OR NEEDLE

Inoculating loops and needles are the most commonly used instruments for transferring microbes between all media types-broths, slants, or plates can be the source and any can be the destination. Since loops and needles are handled in the same way, we refer only to loops in the following instructions for ease of reading.

Obtaining a Sample with an Inoculating Loop or Needle

i. From a Broth

- Suspend bacteria in the broth with a vortex mixer or by agitating the tube with your fingers.
- Flame the loop.
- Remove and hold the tube's cap with little finger of your loop hand.
- Flame the open end of the tube by passing it through a flame two or three times.
- Hold the open tube at an angle to prevent airborne contamination.

- Holding the loop hand still, move the tube up the wire until the tip is in the broth. Continuing to hold the loop hand still, remove the tube from the wire. There should be a film of broth in the loop. Be especially careful not to catch the loop tip on the tube lip. This springing action of the loop creates bacterial aerosols.
- Flame the tube lip as before. Keep your loop hand still.
- Keeping the loop hand still (remember, it has growth on it), move the tube to replace its cap.
- What you do next depends on the medium to which you are transferring the growth. Please continue with appropriate inoculation section.

ii. From a Slant
- Flame the loop.
- Remove and hold the culture tube's cap with the little finger of your loop hand.
- Flame the open end of the tube by passing it through a flame two or three times.
- With the agar surface facing upward, hold the open tube at an angle to prevent airborne contamination.
- Holding the loop hand still, move the tube up the wire until the wire tip is over the desired growth. Touch the loop to the growth and obtain the smallest visible mass of bacteria. Then, holding the loop hand still, remove the tube from the wire. Be especially careful not to catch the loop tip on the tube lip. This springing action of the loop creates bacterial aerosols.
- The Vortex Mixer: Bacteria are suspended in a broth with a vortex mixer. Caution must be used to prevent broth from getting into the cap or losing control of the tube and causing a spill.
- Mixing by Hand: A broth culture should always be mixed prior to transfer. Tapping the tube with your fingers gets the job done safely and without special equipment.
- Use the Lid as a Shield: When transferring bacteria to or from a Petri dish, keep the agar surface covered with the lid to minimize airborne contamination.
- A Loop and Broth: Hold the open tube on an angle to minimize airborne contamination. When placing a loop into a broth tube or removing it, keep the loop hand still and move the tube. Be careful not to catch the loop on the tube's lip when removing it. This produces aerosols that can be dangerous or produce contamination.
- Flame the tube lip as before. Keep your loop hand still.
- Keeping the loop hand still (remember, it has growth on it), move the tube to replace its cap.
- What you do next depends on the medium to which you are transferring the growth. Please continue with the appropriate inoculation section.

iii. From an Agar Plate

- Flame the loop
- Lift the lid of agar plate, but continue to use it as a cover to prevent contamination from above.
- Touch the loop to an uninoculated portion of the plate to cool it. (Placing a hot wire on growth may cause spattering of the growth and create aerosols.) Obtain a small amount of bacterial growth by gently touching a colony with the wire tip.
- Carefully remove the loop from the plate and hold it still as you replace the lid.
- What you do next depends on the medium to which you are transferring the growth. Please continue with the appropriate inoculation section. Inoculation of Media with an Inoculating Loop or Needle.
- Fishtail Inoculation of Agar Slants.
- Agar slants are generally used for growing stock cultures that can be refrigerated after incubation and maintained for several weeks. Many differential media used in identification of microbes are also slants.
- Remove the cap of the sterile medium with little finger of your loop hand and hold it there.
- Flame the tube by quickly passing it through the flame a couple of times. Keep your loop hand still.
- Hold the open tube on an angle to minimize airborne contamination. Keep your loop hand still.
- With the agar surface facing upward, carefully move the tube over the wire. Gently touch the loop to the agar surface near the base.
- Beginning at the bottom of the exposed agar surface, drag the loop in a zigzag pattern as the tube is withdrawn. Be careful not to cut the agar surface and be especially careful not to catch the loop tip on the tube lip as you remove it. This springing action of the loop creates bacterial aerosols.
- Flame the tube mouth as before. Keep your loop hand still.
- Keeping the loop hand still (remember, it has growth on it), move the tube to replace its cap.
- Replacing the Cap: Keeping the loop hand still (remember it has growth on it), move the tube to replace the cap. The cap doesn't have to be on firmly at this point-just enough to cover the tube.
- A Loop and an Agar Slant: When placing a loop into a slant tube or removing it, keep the loop hand still and move the tube. Hold the tube so the agar is facing upwards.
- Fishtail Inoculation of a Slant: Begin at the base of the slant surface and gently move the loop back and forth as you withdraw the tube. Be careful not to cut the agar. Sterilize the loop upon completion of the transfer.

- Sterilize the loop as before by incinerating it in the Bunsen burner flame. It is especially important to flame it from base to tip now because the loop has lots of bacteria on it.
- Label the tube with your name, date and organism. Incubate at the appropriate temperature for the assigned time.

Inoculation of Broth Tubes

Broth cultures are often used to grow cultures for use when fresh cultures or large numbers of cells are desired. Many differential media are also broths.

- Remove the cap of sterile medium with little finger of your loop hand and hold it there.
- Sterilize the tube by quickly passing it through the flame a couple of times. Keep your loop hand still.
- Hold the open tube on an angle to minimize airborne contamination. Keep your loop hand still.
- Carefully move the broth tube over the wire. Gently swirl the loop in the broth to dislodge microbes.
- Withdraw the tube from over the loop. Before completely removing it, touch the loop tip to the glass to remove any excess broth. Then be especially careful not to catch the loop tip on the tube lip when withdrawing it. This springing action of the wire creates bacterial aerosols.
- Inoculation of a Broth: When entering or leaving the tube, move the tube keep the loop hand still. Gently swirl the loop in the broth to transfer the organisms.
- Remove excess broth from loop: Before removing it from the tube, touch the loop to the glass to remove excess broth. Failure to do so will result in splattering and aerosols when sterilizing the loop in a flame.
- Flame the tube lip as before. Keep your loop hand still.
- Keeping the loop hand still (remember, it has growth on it), move the tube to replace its cap.
- Sterilize the loop as before by incinerating it in the Bunsen burner flame. It is especially important to flame it from base to tip now because the loop and wire have lots of bacteria on them.
- Label the tube with your name, date and organism. Incubate at the appropriate temperature for the assigned time.

■ STAINING

Because microbial cytoplasm is usually transparent, it is necessary to stain microorganisms before they can be viewed with light microscope. In some cases, staining is unnecessary, for example, when microorganisms are very large or when motility is to be studied and a drop of the microorganisms can be placed directly on the slide and observed. A preparation like this is called a wet mount.

In preparation for staining, a small sample of microorganism is placed on a slide and permitted to air dry. The smear is heat fixed by quickly passing it over a flame. Heat fixing kills the organisms, makes them adhere to the slide and permits them to accept the stain.

Simple stain techniques (Figure 15.11)

Staining can be performed with basic dyes such as crystal violet or Methylene blue, positively charged dyes that are attracted to the negatively charged materials of the microbial cytoplasm. Such a procedure is the simple stain procedure. An alternative is to use a dye such as Nigrosin or Congo red, acidic, negatively charged dyes. They are repelled by negatively charged cytoplasm and gather around the cells, leaving the cells clear and unstained. This technique is called the negative Stain technique.

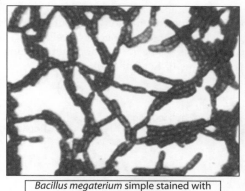

Bacillus megaterium simple stained with methylene blue (1,000 x)

Figure 15.11: Simple stained *Bacillus Megaterium* with methylene blue

Differential stain techniques

Differential staining techniques help to differentiate two different types of organisms. Example: Gram Staining Technique. This technique helps to separate bacteria into two groups such as Gram positive bacteria and Gram negative bacteria.

Gram Staining Technique

Although simple stains are useful, they do not reveal details about the bacteria other than morphology and arrangement. The Gram stain is a differential stain commonly used in the microbiology laboratory that differentiates bacteria on the basis of their cell wall structure. Most bacteria can be divided into two groups based on the composition of their cell wall:

Principle:

▪ Gram-positive cell walls have a thick peptidoglycan layer beyond the plasma membrane. Characteristic polymers called Teichoic and Lipoteichoic acids stick out above the peptidoglycan and it is because of their negative charge that the cell wall is overall negative. These acids are also very important in the body's ability to recognize foreign bacteria. Gram-positive cell walls stain blue/purple with the Gram stain.

▪ Gram-negative cell walls are more complex. They have a thin peptidoglycan layer and an outer membrane beyond the plasma membrane. The space between the plasma membrane and the outer membrane is called as the periplasmic space. The outer leaflet of the outer membrane is largely composed of a molecule called Lipopolysaccharide (LPS). Lipopolysaccharide is an endotoxin that is important in triggering the body's immune response and contributing to the overall negative charge of the cell. Spanning the outer membrane are porin proteins that enable the passage of small molecules. Lipoproteins join the outer membrane and the thin peptidoglycan layer. Gram-negative cells will stain pink with the Gram stain. This is the most important staining technique in Bacteriology (Figures 15.12 (A and B)).

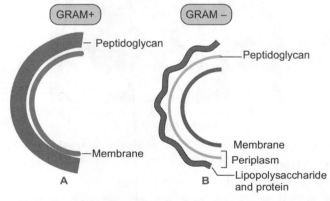

Figures 15.12 (A and B): The cell wall of (A) Gram-Positive Bacteria showing peptidoglycan layer and (B) Gram-Negative Bacteria showing lipopolysaccharide layer over peptidoglycan layer

Steps of Gram Staining

▪ Place a slide with a bacterial smear on a staining rack.
▪ **STAIN** the slide with Crystal Violet for 1-2 min.
▪ Pour off the stain.
   Note: fingers stain Gram-positive - use forceps!
▪ Flood slide with Gram's iodine for 1-2 min.

- Pour off the Iodine.
- Decolourize by washing the slide briefly with Acetone for (2-3 seconds).
- Wash slide thoroughly with water to remove the Acetone - do not delay this step.
- Flood slide with Safranin counterstain for 2 min.
- Wash with water.
- Blot excess water and dry in hand over bunsen flame.

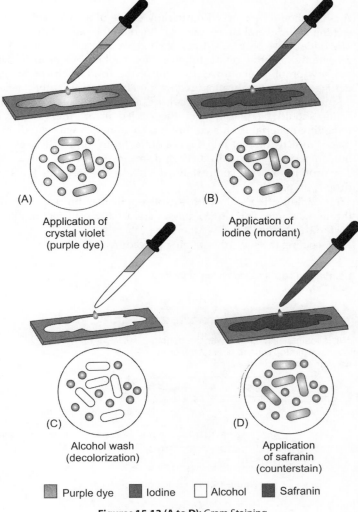

(A) Application of crystal violet (purple dye)

(B) Application of iodine (mordant)

(C) Alcohol wash (decolorization)

(D) Application of safranin (counterstain)

■ Purple dye   ■ Iodine   ☐ Alcohol   ■ Safranin

Figures 15.13 (A to D): Gram Staining

■ PREPARATION OF SLIDE

A properly prepared smear accomplishes two things. It causes bacteria to adhere to a slide so that they can be stained and observed. It also kills them, rendering pathogenic bacteria safe to handle. An objective in preparing smears is to learn to recognize the correct density of bacteria to place on the slide. Too much of overlapping gives false positives or crowd each other to make a mess. A few of it cannot be located on the slide.

- A circle should be marked on the underside of a slide with a glass etching tool. Several circles can be located on the same slide.
- The slide must be grease-free. A good way to clean a slide is to repeatedly breathe on it followed by rubbing vigorously with a Kimwipe or paper towel to remove the fog. When the slide is defogged immediately after breathing on it, it is sufficiently cleaned.
- To prepare a smear from a dry culture, a very small drop of distilled water should be placed over the circled area. After aseptically removing material from a culture it is them mixed with the drop or placed directly on the slide if it is a dilute broth culture. It takes very little material to produce a successful smear.
- The drop is air-dried completely which takes a short time if a small drop is prepared.
- While holding the slide with a clothes pin it is quickly passed it through a flame. Three quick passes are usually sufficient to kill the bacteria and cause them to adhere.
- After cooling the slide, the staining procedure is conducted.

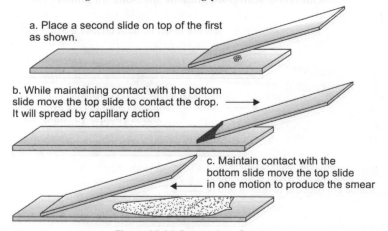

a. Place a second slide on top of the first as shown.

b. While maintaining contact with the bottom slide move the top slide to contact the drop. → It will spread by capillary action

c. Maintain contact with the bottom slide move the top slide in one motion to produce the smear

Figure 15.14: Preparation of smear

Direct Stain

Microbial cells are small and transparent. Stains are often used to increase contrast between the cells and the background, making them easier to see under the microscope. Since many of the cell components are negatively charged, stains with positively charged chromophores (the colored ion of the dye) will attach to the cells. Examples of such stains include Methylene blue, Crystal violet and Carbon Fuschin.

- Make a heat-fixed smear, taking care not to use too much culture if working from an agar culture.
- Place the slide on a staining rack over a sink or catch basin.
- Add a drop of dye to the smear. You need enough stain to just cover the smear, not the whole slide.
- Allow the dye to act. (One minute is generally adequate.)
- Gently rinse the dye from the slide with water from a squirt bottle.
- Gently blot the slide and observe under the microscope.

Fixation

The process by which the internal and external structures of micro-organisms are preserved and fixed in place is called Fixation.

- Heat fixation: Fixation by means of application of heat. The prepared smear of microorganisms is gently heated and dried.
- Chemical fixation: It involves the use of chemicals such as ethanol and Formaldehyde.

■ EXAMINATION OF SLIDE

Methods by which you can examine culture slides which include the following:

- Staining
- Microscopy

Staining

Because microbial cytoplasm is usually transparent, it is necessary to stain microorganisms before they can be viewed with light microscope. In some cases, staining is unnecessary, for example when microorganisms are very large or when motility is to be studied and a drop of microorganisms can be placed directly on the slide and observed. A preparation such as this is called a wet mount. A wet mount can also be prepared by placing a drop of culture on a cover slip (a glass cover for a slide) and then inverting it over a hollowed out slide. This procedure is called the hanging drop.

In preparation for staining, a small sample of microorganisms is placed on a slide and permitted to air dry. The smear is heat fixed by quickly passing it over a flame. Heat fixing kills the organisms, makes them adhere to the slide and permits them to accept the stain.

Applications of Staining:

1. Used to increase visibility of microorganisms being studied.
2. Used to identify the shape of bacteria.
3. Used to determine the morphological features of microorganisms.
4. Used to detect contamination.
5. Used to differentiate and classify microorganisms (differential stains).
6. Used to detect bacterial parts such as capsule, spores, flagella or inclusion bodies (special stains).

Microscopy

What is a Microscope?

To view microscopic organisms, their magnification is essential. The microscope is the instrument used to magnify microscopic images. Its function and some aspects of design are similar to those of telescopes although the microscope is designed to visualize very small close objects while telescope magnifies distant objects.

Types of Microscope (Figure: 15.15)

Depending on the working principle, construction and mode of functioning microscope is of two types;

1. Light Microscope – which functions in the presence of light rays. It is of following types;

(a) Bright-field Microscope,

(b) Dark-field Microscope,

(c) Phase-contrast Microscope,

(d) Differential Interference Contrast (DIC) Microscope,

(e) Fluorescence Microscope

2. Electron Microscope – Which functions in the presence of beam of electrons. It is of following types ;

(a) Scanning Electron Microscope

(b) Transmission Electron Microscope

The Light Microscope

The Bright-Field Microscope is the most common type of light microscope found in the microbiology diagnostic laboratories. We will discuss that in detail.

i. Working Principle

Basically, a light microscope magnifies small objects and makes them visible. The science of microscopy is based on the following concepts and principles:

Magnification is simply the enlargement of the specimen. In a compound lens system, each lens sequentially enlarges or magnifies the specimen. The **objective lens** magnifies the specimen, producing a **real image** that is then magnified by the **occular lens** resulting in the final image. The **total magnification** can be calculated by multiplying the objective lens value by the occular lens value.

Resolving power is the ability of a lens to show two adjacent objects as discrete entities.

Limit of Resolution is the ability to see two closely placed dots as two separate dots. If the distance between the two points is lessened, it would appear as a single point. It is expressed quantitatively as limit of resolution. The resolution of human unaided eye is 200 mμ.

Numerical Aperture of the lens decides the angle at which the light enters it. The light-gathering ability of a microscope objective lens is quantitatively expressed in terms of numerical aperture.

Contrast is the ability to distinguish an object from its background. Since most microbes are relatively transparent when viewed under a standard light microscope they are difficult to identify. Using a stain that will bind to the microorganism and not the glass slide, enhances their contrast enabling them to be observed more clearly.

Depth-of-focus is the "thickness" of the sample that appears in focus at a particular magnification. As the magnification increases the depth-of-focus decreases or the "slice" of the sample that appears in focus gets thinner.

Field-of-View is the area of the slide that you are observing through the microscope. As you increase the magnification the actual area of the slide that you are looking at is getting smaller.

Working distance is the distance between the objective and the slide. As you increase magnification (by using more powerful objective lenses) the working distance decreases.

ii. Construction

Eyepiece: contains the ocular lens, which provides a magnification power of 10 to 15, usually. This is where you look through.

Nosepiece: holds the objective lenses and can be rotated easily to change magnification.

Objective lenses: usually, there are three or four objective lenses on a microscope, consisting of 4×, 10×, 40× and 100× magnification powers. In order to obtain the total magnification of an image, you need to multiply the eyepiece lens power by the objective lens power. So, if you couple a 10 eyepiece lens with a 40x objective lens, the total magnification is of 10×40 = 400 times.

Stage clips: hold the slide in place.

Stage: it is a flat platform that supports the slide being analyzed.

Diaphragm: it controls the intensity and size of the cone light projected on the specimen. As a rule of thumb, the more transparent the specimen, less light is required.

Light source: it projects light upwards through the diaphragm, slide and lenses.

Base: supports the microscope.

Condenser lens: it helps to focus the light onto the sample analyzed. They are particularly helpful when coupled with the highest objective lens.

Arm: supports the microscope when carried.

Coarse adjustment knob: when the knob is turned, the stage moves up or down, in order to coarse adjust the focus.

Fine adjustment knob: used fine adjust the focus.

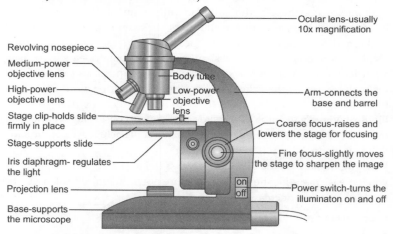

Figure 15. 15: Parts of a bright field compound microscope used in microbiology laboratories

Handling and Care

▪ Use two hands when carrying a microscope, be gentle, these are sensitive and expensive instruments. Keep the microscope upright, oculars are removable and could fall out.

▪ Clean or dry lenses with grit-free lens paper only. Booklets of it are on your table's tray.

▪ Never use anything but lens paper. Other papers, tissues, or cloth will scratch lenses.

▪ Keep eyepiece (s) in the microscope at all times to keep dust out of the tube.

▪ Do not unscrew or otherwise tamper with lenses unless instructed to do so.

▪ At the start, do not look into the microscope. Begin by raising the stage as high as it can go by turning the coarse focal knob. You can now look through the ocular and focus on the specimen by turning the focus knob very slowly, in one direction.

- To change the magnification, grasp the ring of the revolving nosepiece and rotate until the desired objective clicks into place. Do not use the objectives to turn the nose-piece.
- Each time you complete work, particularly with oil immersion, clean the lenses with lens paper. Clean oil and other liquids from the stage and table as well.
- When you have finished with the microscope.
- The lowest power objective (it is also the shortest one) or none, should be returned to the position of use, before removing the slide.
- The slide is removed from stage and cleaned by rinsing in ethanol, unless it is a prepared slide, then it should go back onto a slide tray.
- The lenses and stage should be clean and dry. The cord loosely wrapped about the arm.
- The ocular rotated so it faces the back of the scope. (As not hit the back wall of the cabinet when returned to the shelf.)

Uses: These microscopes are used by laboratories, universities and hospitals to look at biological specimens for research and diagnostics.

Advantages:
- Brightfield microscopy is very simple to use with fewer adjustments needed to be made to view specimens.
- Some specimens can be viewed without staining and the technology used in the brightfield technique don't alter the color of the specimen.

Limitations
- Brightfield microscopy can't be used to observe living specimens of bacteria, although when using fixed specimens, bacteria have an optimum viewing magnification of 1000x.
- Brightfield microscopy has very low contrast and most cells absolutely have to be stained to be seen. Staining may introduce extra details into the specimen that should not be present.
- This method requires a strong light source for high magnification applications and intense lighting can produce heat that will damage specimens or kill living microorganisms.

■ POSSIBLE QUESTIONS

1. Describe the methods of isolating pure cultures with necessary diagrams.
2. Write in detail about the culture media with its classification.
3. What are the types of culture media?
4. Describe what are the different methods of preparing culture slides? Explain fixation.

5. What are the different staining methods and explain each of them with necessary examples?
6. What is a microscope and describe its structure with diagram?
7. Describe the types of microscopes in detail.
8. Explain the following:
   - Aseptic transfer
   - Inoculation from a broth
   - Inoculation from a slant
   - Negative staining
   - Gram Staining
   - Method of inoculation
   - Inoculation of culture media
   - Culture Media
   - Subculturing
   - Isolation of Microorganisms
   - Streak Plate and Pour Plate
   - Selective and enrichment media
   - Differential Media

Model Questions and Answers

1. Give a detail account of the bacterial cell.

Answer

- **Introduction-** Bacteria are microscopic, prokaryotic, unicellular organisms which are found everywhere.
- **Ultrastructure of Bacterial Cell-**

Followings are the parts of a bacterial cell;

(a) Capsule and slime layer

- **Location:** Outermost covering of the bacterial cell.
- **Structure:** Polysaccharide layers can be thick and stable like capsule or loosely attached to cell wall like slime layer.
- **Function:** Assist cells in adhesion to solid surface, and also protect pathogenic bacteria from the attack of the host's immune system.

(b) Cell wall

- **Location:** It is present next to the capsule or slime layer.
- **Structure:** It is mostly composed of Peptidoglycan. In Gram-positive bacteria the peptidoglcan layer is thicker and contains techoic acid, whereas in Gram-negative bacteria the peptidoglycan layer is thinner and contains lipopolysaccharide.
- **Function:** It protects the cell from osmotic shock and physical damage. It also provides rigidity and shape to bacterial cells.

(c) Cell membrane

- **Location:** Next to cell wall.
- **Structure:** The cell membrane is made up of Phospholipid bilayer, having thickness of 6-8 nm. A phospholipid molecule consists of one hydrophilic phosphate group and two hydrophobic Fatty acid chains.

Hydrophillic heads are exposed to the external environments or the cytoplasm. The fatty acid chains direct inward, facing each other due to hydrophobic effects.

- **Function:** Regulates the specific transport of substances between the cells and the outer environment.

(d) Cytoplasm

- **Location:** Present inside the cell.
- **Composition:** It is a semifluid substance enclosed by the cell membrane. It appears granular due to the presence of large number of ribosomes. Different structures such as chromosomes, plasmids as well as cytoplasmic organelles are found in the cytoplasm.
- **Function:** It is the site for various biochemical reactions and contains genetic material of the cell.

(e) Chromosome

This is also called as Nucleoid.

- **Location:** Found to float freely in the cytoplasm.
- **Number:** One chromosome in each cell.
- **Size:** In E. coli the size of chromosome is 4640 kilo base pairs (kbp).
- **Structure & Composition:** It is made up of circular DNA attached at a point to the plasma membrane. The DNA in bacterial cell is not associated with histone protein. The DNA molecule is composed of Nitrogen Bases (A,T,G,C), deoxyribose sugar and phosphate molecules.
- **Function:** It is the storehouse of genetic information.

Note: Apart from the Nucleoid, some bacterial cells also contain plasmids.

(f) Ribosomes

- **Location:** It is evenly distributed in the cytoplasm.
- **Structure and Composition:** Bacteria contain 70S Ribosome made up of ribosomal RNA (rRNA) and proteins. 70S Ribosome has two subunits (30S and 50S).
- **Function:** They are involved in bacterial protein synthesis

(g) Locomotory organs

They are of two types- Flagella and Cilia.

- **Location:** Outer most part of the cell.
- **Structure:** Flagella are made of flagellin proteins.
- **Function:** The primary function of flagella is to make the bacteria move.

(h) Inclusion bodies

- **Location:** Distributed in the cytoplasm.
- They are the non-living components present in the cell which do not possess metabolic activity. The most common inclusion bodies are glycogen, lipid droplets, crystals, pigments, volutin granules and metachromatic granules.

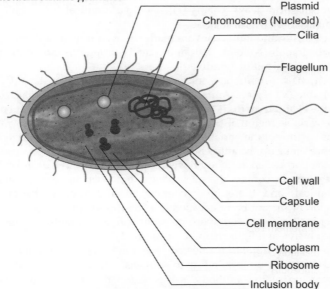

Figure 1: Ultra Structure of a bacterial cell

2. Write Short Notes:

(a) Koch's Postulates

Answer: Koch's postulates are criteria designed to establish a relationship between a microbe and a disease. The postulates were published by Koch in 1890. Followings are the Koch's postulates;

- A specific organism should be found constantly in association with the disease.
- The organism should be isolated and grown in a pure culture in the laboratory.
- The pure culture when inoculated into a healthy susceptible animal should produce symptoms/lesions of the same disease.
- From the inoculated animal, the microorganism should be isolated in pure culture.

- An additional criterion introduced is that specific anitbodies to the causative organism should be demonstrable in patient's serum.
- Significance: They tell us how to definitively prove that a particular microbe causes a given disease.

(b) Structure of Antibody

- It is a "Y"-shaped molecule that consists of four polypeptide chains; two identical heavy chains (H) and two identical light chains (L) connected by disulfide bonds
- Each heavy and light chain are made up of a number of domains .
- Each domain is about 110 amino acids in length and contains an interchain disulfide bond.
- Each chain in antibody consists of two regions- Constant (C) and Variable (V) region. Amino acid sequence in the C-terminal regions of the H and L chains is the same whereas the amino acid sequence in the variable region of H and L chains is different.
- The regions of the variable domains actually contact the antigen and hence make up the antigen-binding site.
- Some parts of an antibody have unique functions. The arms of the Y, for example, contain the sites that can bind two antigens (in general identical) and therefore, recognize specific foreign objects. This region of the antibody is called the Fab (fragment, antigen binding) region. It is composed of one constant and one variable domain from each heavy and light chain of the antibody
- The variable domain is referred to as the FV region and is the most important region for binding to antigens.
- Fc region of the antibody is the region that trigger complement fixation reaction.

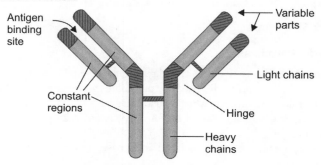

Figure 2: Structure of antibody

(c) Pasteurization

- This is a special technique of heat sterilization developed by Louis Pasteur.
- Originally it was used to kill undesirable microorganisms that cause souring of wine
- This process was originally employed by Louis Pasteur.
- Currently this procedure is employed in food and dairy industry.
- There are three methods of pasteurization,
  - Holder method -Heated at 63°C for 30 minutes
  - Flash method -Heated at 72°C for 15 seconds followed by quickly cooling to 13°C
  - Ultra-High Temperature (UHT)-140°C for 15 sec and 149°C for 0.5 sec.
- This method is suitable to destroy most milk borne pathogens like *Salmonella*, *Mycobacteria*, *Streptococci*, *Staphylococci* and *Brucella*.
- However, *Coxiella* may survive pasteurization.

(d) Gram Staining

Objective: To differentiate between Gram-positive and Gram-negative bacteria.

Requirements: Glass slide, microbial culture, inoculation loop, Bunsen burner, Crystal violet, Ethanol, Safranin, Distilled water, Blotting paper, Light microscope.

Methodology:

- Place a slide with a bacterial smear on a staining rack.
- Stain the slide with Crystal Violet for 1-2 min.
- Pour off the stain.
- Flood slide with Gram's iodine for 1-2 min.
- Pour off the iodine.
- Decolourize by washing the slide briefly with acetone for 2-3 seconds.
- Wash slide thoroughly with water to remove the acetone - do not delay this step.
- Flood slide with Safranin counter stain for 2 min.
- Wash with water.
- Blot excess water and dry in hand over bunsen flame.
- Observe it under the Microscope.

Inference: Bacteria with blue stain are Gram-positive where as bacteria with red stain are Gram-negative.

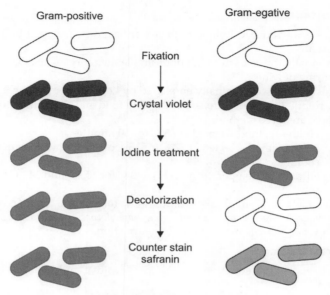

Figure 3: Steps of gram staining

Glossary

1. AB Toxins: The structure and activity of many exotoxins are based on the AB model. In this model, the B portion of the toxin is responsible for toxin binding to a cell but does not directly harm it. The A portion enters the cell and disrupts its function.

2. Accessory Pigments: Photosynthetic pigments such as carotenoids and phycobiliproteins that aid chlorophyll in trapping light energy.

3. Acid Fast: Refers to bacteria like the mycobacteria that cannot be easily decolorized with acid alcohol after being stained with dyes such as basic fuchsin.

4. Acid-Fast Staining: A staining procedure that differentiates between bacteria based on their ability to retain a dye when washed with an acid alcohol solution.

5. Acidophile: A microorganism that has its growth optimum between about pH 0 and 5.5

6. Acquired Immune Deficiency Syndrome (AIDS): An infectious disease syndrome caused by the human immunodeficiency virus and is characterized by the loss of a normal immune response, followed by increased susceptibility to opportunistic infections and an increased risk of some cancers.

7. Acquired Immune Tolerance: The ability to produce antibodies against nonself antigens while "tolerating" (not producing antibodies against) self-antigens.

8. Acquired Immunity: Refers to the type of specific (adaptive) immunity that develops after exposure to a suitable antigen or is produced after antibodies are transferred from one individual to another.

9. Actinobacteria: A group of Gram-positive bacteria containing the actinomycetes and their high G + C relatives.

10. Actinomycete: An aerobic, Gram-positive bacterium that forms branching filaments (hyphae) and asexual spores.

11. Actinorhizae: Associations between actinomycetes and plant roots.

12. Activated Sludge: Solid matter or sediment composed of actively growing microorganisms that participate in the aerobic portion of a biological sewage treatment process. The microbes readily use dissolved organic substrates and transform them into additional microbial cells and carbon dioxide.

13. Active Immunization: The induction of active immunity by natural exposure to a pathogen or by vaccination.

14. Acute Infections: Virus infections with a fairly rapid onset that last for a relatively short time.

15. Acute Viral Gastroenteritis: An inflammation of the stomach and intestines, normally caused by Norwalk and Norwalklike viruses, other caliciviruses, rotaviruses and astroviruses.

16. Adenine: A purine derivative, 6-aminopurine, found in nucleosides, nucleotides, coenzymes and nucleic acids.

17. Adenosine Diphosphate (ADP): The nucleoside diphosphate usually formed upon the breakdown of ATP when it provides enregy for work.

18. Adenosine 5'-triphosphate (ATP): The triphosphate of the nucleoside adenosine, which is a high energy molecule or has high phosphate group transfer potential and serves as the cell's major form of energy currency.

19. Adhesin: A molecular component on the surface of a microorganism that is involved in adhesion to a substratum or cell. Adhesion to a specific host issue usually is a preliminary stage in pathogenesis, and adhesins are important virulence factors.

20. Adjuvant: Material added to an antigen to increase its immunogenicity. Common examples are alum, killed Bordetella pertussis, and an oil emulsion of the antigen, either alone (Freund's incomplete adjuvant) or with killed mycobacteria (Freund's complete adjuvant).

21. Aerobe: An organism that grows in the presence of atmospheric oxygen.

22. Aerobic Anoxygenic Photosynthesis: Photosynthetic process in which electron donors such as organic matter or sulfide, which do not result in oxygen evolution, are used under aerobic conditions.

23. Aerobic Respiration: A metabolic process in which molecules, often organic, are oxidized with oxygen as the final electron acceptor.

24. Aerotolerant Anaerobes: Microbes that grow equally well whether or not oxygen is present.

25. Aflatoxin: A polyketide secondary fungal metabolite that can cause cancer.

26. Agar: A complex sulfated polysaccharide, usually from red algae, that is used as a solidifying agent in the preparation of culture media.

27. Agglutinates: The visible aggregates or clumps formed by an agglutination reaction.

28. Agglutination Reaction: The formation of an insoluble immune complex by the cross-linking of cells or particles.

29. Airborne Transmission: The type of infectious organism transmission in which the pathogen is truly suspended in the air and travels over a meter or more from the source to the host.

30. Alkinetes: Specialized, nonmotile, dormant, thick-walled resting cells formed by some cyanobacteria.

31. Alga: A common term for a series of unrelated groups of photosynthetic eucaryotic microorganisms lacking multicellular sex organs (except for the charophytes) and conducting vessels.

32. Algicide: An agent that kills algae.

33. Alkalophile: A microorganism that grows best at pHs from about 8.5 to 11.5.

34. Allergen: A substance capable of inducing allergy or specific susceptibility.

35. Alpha Hemolysis: A greenish zone of partial clearing around a bacteria colony growing on blood agar.

36. Alpha-proteobacteria: One of the five subgroups of proteobacteria, each with distinctive 16S rRNA sequences. This group contains most of the oligotrophic proteobacteria; some have unusual metabolic modes such as methylotrophy, chemolithotrophy, and nitrogen fixing ability. Many have distinctive morphological features.

37. Alveolar Macrophage: A vigorously phagocytic macrophage located on the epithelial surface of the lung alveoli where it ingests inhaled particulate matter and microorganisms.

38. Amensalism: A relationship in which the product of one organism has a negative effect on another organism.

39. Ames Test: A test that uses a special Salmonella strain to test chemicals for mutagenicity and potential carcinogenicity.

40. Amino Acid Activation: The initial stage of protein synthesis in which amino acids are attached to transfer RNA molecules.

41. Aminoglycoside Antibiotics: A group of antibiotics synthesized by Streptomyces and Micromonospora, which contain a cyclohexane ring and amino sugars; all aminoglycoside antibiotics bind to the small ribosomal subunit and inhibit protein synthesis.

42. Amphibolic Pathways: Metabolic pathways that function both catabolically and anabolically.

43. Amphitrichous: A cell with a single flagellum at each end.

44. Amphotericin B: An antibiotic from a strain of Streptomyces nodosus that is used to treat systemic fungal infections; it also is used topically to treat candidiasis.

45. Anaerobe: An organism that grows in the absence of free oxygen.

46. Anaerobic Digestion: The microbiological treatment of sewage wastes under anaerobic conditions to produce methane.

47. Anaerobic Respiration: An erergy-yielding process in which the electron transport chain acceptor is an inorganic molecule other than oxygen.

48. Anammox Process: The coupled use of nitrite as an electron acceptor and ammonium ion as a donor under anaerobic conditions to yield nitrogen gas.

49. Anaphylaxis: An immediate (type I) hypersensitivity reaction following exposure of a sensitized individual to the appropriate antigen. Mediated by reagin antibodies, chiefly IgE.

50. Anthrax: An infectious disease of animals caused by ingesting Bacillus anthracis spores. Can also occur in humans and is sometimes called woolsorter's disease.

51. Antibiotic: A microbial product or its derivative that kills susceptible microorganisms or inhibits their growth.

52. Antimetabolite: A compound that blocks metabolic pathways function by competitively inhibiting a key enzyme's use of a metabolite because it closely resembles the normal enzyme substrate.

53. Antimicrobial Agent: An agent that kills microorganisms or inhibits their growth.

54. Antisepsis: The prevention of infection or sepsis.

55. Antiseptic: Chemical agents applied to tissue to prevent infection by killing or inhibiting pathogens.

56. Antitoxin: An antibody to a microbial toxin, usually a bacterial exotoxin, that combines specifically with the toxin, in vivo and in vitro, neutralizing the toxin.

57. Apoptosis: Programmed cell death. The fragmentation of a cell into membrane-bound particles that are eliminated by phagocytosis. Apoptosis is a physiological suicide mechanism that preserves homeostasis and occurs during normal tissue turnover. It causes cell death in pathological circumstances, such as exposure to low concentrations of xenobiotics and infections by HIV and various other viruses.

58. Artificially Acquired Active Immunity: The type of immunity that results from immunizing an animal with a vaccine. The immunized animal now produces its own antibodies and activated lymphocytes.

59. Artificially Acquired Passive Immunity: The type of immunity that results from introducing into an animal antibodies that have been produced either in another animal or by in vitro methods. Immunity is only temporary.

60. Ascocarp: A multicellular structure in ascomycetes lined with specialized cells called asci in which nuclear fusion and meiosis produce ascospores. An ascocarp can be open or closed and may be referred to as a fruiting body.

61. Ascogenous Hypha: A specialized hypha that gives rise to one or more asci.

62. Ascomycetes: A division of fungi that form ascospores.

63. Ascus: A specialized cell, characteristic of the ascomycetes, in which two haploid nuclei fuse to produce a zygote, which immediately divides by meiosis; at maturity an ascus will contain ascospores.

64. Aspergillosis: A fungal disease caused by species of Aspergillus.

65. Atomic Force Microscope: A type of scanning probe microscope that images a surface by moving a sharp probe over the surface at a constant distance : a very small amount of force is exerted on the tip and probe movement is followed with a laser.

66. Attenuation: (1) A mechanism for the regulation of transcription of some bacterial operons by aminoacyl-tRNAs. (2) A procedure that reduces or abolishes the virulence of a pathogen without altering its immunogenicity.

67. Attenuator: A rho-independent termination site in the leader sequence that is involved in attenuation.

68. Autoclave: An apparatus for sterilizing objects by the use of steam under pressure. Its development tremendously stimulated the growth of microbiology.

69. Autogenous Infection: An infection that results from a patient's own microbiota, regardless of whether the infecting organism became part of the patient's microbiota subsequent to admission to a clinical care facility.

70. Autoimmune Disease: A disease produced by the immune system attacking self-antigens. Autoimmune disease results from the activation of self-reactive T and B cells that damage tissues after stimulation by genetic or environmental triggers.

71. Autoimmunity: Autoimmunity is a condition characterized by the presence of serum autoantibodies and self-reactive lymphocytes. It may be benign or pathogenic. Autoimmunity is a normal consequence of aging ; is readily inducible by infectious agents, organisms, or drugs ; and is potentially reversible in that it disappears when the offending "agent" is removed or eradicated.

72. Autotroph: An organism that uses CO_2 as its sole or principal source of carbon.

73. Auxotroph: A mutated prototroph that lacks the ability to synthesize an essen'ial nutrient and therefore, must obtain it or a precursor from its surroundings.

74. Axenic: Not contaminated by any foreign organisms; the term is used in reference to pure microbial cultures or to germfree animals.

75. Bacillus: A rod-shaped bacterium.

76. Bacteremia: The presence of viable bacteria in the blood.

77. Bacteria: The domain that contains procaryotic cells with primarily diacyl glycerol diesters in their membranes and with bacterial rRNA. Bacteria also is a general term for organisms that are composed of procaryotic cells and are not multicellular.

78. **Bacterial Artificial Chromosome (BAC):** A cloning vector constructed from the E. coli F-factor plasmid that is used to clone foreign DNA fragments in E. coli.

79. **Bacterial Vaginosis:** Bacterial vaginosis is a sexually trasmitted disease caused by Gardnerella vaginalis, Mobiluncus spp., Mycoplasma hominis, and various anaerobic bacteria. Although a mild disease it is a risk factor for obstetric infections and pelvic inflammatory disease.

80. **Bactericide:** An agent that kills bacteria.

81. **Bacteriochlorophyll:** A modified chlorophyll that serves as the primary light-trapping pigment in purple and green photosynthetic bacteria.

82. **Bacteriocin:** A protein produced by a bacterial strain that kills other closely related strains.

83. **Bacteriophage:** A virus that uses bacteria as its host; often called a phage.

84. **Bacteriophage (phage) Typing:** A technique in which strains of bacteria are identified based on their susceptibility to bacteriophages.

85. **Bacteriostatic:** Inhibiting the growth and reproduction of bacteria.

86. **Bacteroid:** A modified, often pleomorphic, bacterial cell within the root nodule cells of legumes; after transformation into a symbiosome it carries out nitrogen fixation.

87. **Baeocytes:** Small, spherical, reproductive cells produced by pleurocapsalean cyanobacteria through multiple fission.

88. **Balanced Growth:** Microbial growth in which all cellular constituents are synthesized at constant rates relative to eath other.

89. **Balanitis:** Inflammation of the glans penis usually associated with Candida fungi; a sexually transmitted disease.

90. **Barophilic or Barophile:** Organisms that prefer or require high pressures for growth and reproduction.

91. **Barotolerant:** Organisms that can grow and reproduce at high pressures but do not require them.

92. **Basal Body:** The cylindrical structure at the base of procaryotic and eucaryotic flagella that attaches them to the cell.

93. **Batch Culture:** A culture of microorganisms produced by inoculating a closed culture vessel containing a single batch of medium.

94. **B-cell Antigen Receptor (BCR):** A transmembrane immunoglobulin complex on the surface of a B cell that binds an antigen and stimulates the B cell. It is composed of a membrane-bound immunoglobulin, usually IgD or a modified IgM, complexed with another membrane protein (the Ig-α/Ig-β heterodimer).

95. **Beta Hemolysis:** A zone of complete clearing around a bacterial colony growing on blood agar. The zone does not change significantly in color.

96. β-Oxidation Pathway: The major pathway of fatty acid oxidation to produce NADH, FADH2 and acetyl coenzyme A.

97. Beta-proteobacteria: One of the five subgroups of proteobacteria, each with distinctive 16S rRNA sequences. Members of this subgroup are similar to the alpha-proteobacteria metabolically, but tend to use substances that diffuse from organic matter decomposition in anaerobic zones.

98. Binal Symmetry: The symmetry of some virus capsids (e.g., those of complex phages) that is a combination of icosahedral and helical symmetry.

99. Binary Fission: Asexual reproduction in which a cell or an organism separates into two cells.

100. Bioaugmentation: Addition of pregrown microbial cultures to an environment to perform a specific task.

101. Biochemical Oxygen Demand (BOD): The amount of oxygen used by organisms in water under certain standard conditions; it provides an index of the amount of microbially oxidizable organic matter present.

102. Biodegradation: The breakdown of a complex chemical through biological processes that can result in minor loss of functional groups, fragmentation into larger constituents, or complete breakdown to carbon dioxide and minerals. Often the term refers to the undesired microbialmediated destruction of materials such as paper, paint, and textiles.

103. Biofilms: Organized microbial systems consisting of layers of microbial cells associated with surfaces, often with complex structural and functional characteristics. Biofilms have physical/chemical gradients that influence microbial metabolic processes. They can form on inanimate devices (catheters, medical prosthetic devices) and also cause fouling (e.g., of ships' hulls, water pipes, cooling towers).

104. Biogeochemical Cycling: The oxidation and reduction of substances carried out by living organisms and/or abiotic processes that results in the cycling of elements within and between different parts of the ecosystem (the soil, aquatic environment and atomshpere).

105. Bioinsecticide: A pathogen that is used to kill or disable unwanted insect pests. Bacteria, fungi, or viruses are used, either directly or after manipulation, to control insect populations.

106. Biologic Transmission: A type of vector-borne transmission in which a pathogen goes through some morphological or physiological change within the vector.

107. Bioluminescence: The production of light by living cells, often through the oxidation of molecules by the enzyme luciferase.

108. Biopesticide: The use of a microorganism or another biological agent to control a specific pest.

109. Bioremediation: The use of biologically mediated processes to remove or degrade pollutants from specific environments. Bioremediation can be carried out by modification of the environment to accelerate biological processes, either with or without the addition of specific microorganisms.

110. Biosensor: The coupling of a biological process with production of an electrical signal or light to detect the presence of particular substances.

111. Bioterrorism: The intentional or threatened use of viruses, bacteria, fungi, or toxins from living organisms to produce death or disease in humans, animals, and plants.

112. Biotransformation or Microbial Transformation: The use of living organisms to modify substances that are not normally used for growth.

113. Black Peidra: A fungal infection caused by Piedraia hortae that forms hard black nodules on the hairs of the scalp.

114. Blastomycosis: A systemic fungal infection caused by Blastomyces dermatitidis and marked by suppurating tumors in the skin or by lesions in the lungs.

115. Botulism: A form of food poisoning caused by a neurotoxin (botulin) produced by Clostridium botulinum serotypes A-G; sometimes found in improperly canned or preserved food.

116. Bright-field Microscope: A microscope that illuminates the specimen directly with bright light and forms a dark image on a brighter background.

117. Broad-spectrum Drugs: Chemotherapeutic agents that are effective against many different kinds of pathogens.

118. Budding: A vegetative outgrowth of yeast and some bacteria as a means of asexual reproduction; the daughter cell is smaller than the parent.

119. Bulking Sludge: Sludges produced in sewage treatment that do not settle properly, usually due to the development of filamentous microorganisms.

120. Butanediol Fermentation: A type of fermentation most often found in the family Enterobacteriaceae in which 2, 3-butanediol is a major product; acetoin is an intermediate in the pathway and may be detected by the Voges-Proskauer test.

121. Candidiasis: An infection caused by Candida species of dimorphic fungi, commonly involving the skin.

122. Capsule: A layer of well-organized material, not easily washed off, lying outside the bacterial cell wall.

123. Carboxysomes: Polyhedral inclusion bodies that contain the CO_2 fixation enzyme ribulose 1, 5- bisphosphate carboxylase; found in cyanobacteria, nitrifying bacteria and thiobacilli.

124. Carrier: An infected individual who is a potential source of infection for others and plays an important role in the epidemiology of a disease.

125. Caseous Lesion: A lesion resembling cheese or curd; cheesy. Most caseous lesions are caused by M. tuberculosis.

126. Casual Carrier: An individual who harbors an infectious organism for only a short period.

127. Cathelicidins: Antimicrobial peptides that are produced by skin cells and kill bacterial pathogens. They destroy invaders by either punching holes in their membranes or solubilizing membranes through detergent-like action.

128. Cellulitis. A diffuse spreading infection of subcutaneous skin tissue caused by streptococci, staphylococci, or other organisms. The tissue is inflamed with edema, redness, pain, and interference with function.

129. Cell Wall: The strong layer or structure that lies outside the plasma membrane; it supports and protects the membrane and gives the cell shape.

130. Cephalosporin: A group of β-lactam antibiotics derived from the fungus Cephalosporium, which share the 7-aminocephalosporanic acid nucleus.

131. Chancroid: A sexually transmitted disease caused by the Gram-negative bacterium Haemophilus ducreyi. Worldwide, chancroid is an important cofactor in the transmission of the AIDS virus. Also known as genital ulcer disease due to the painful circumscribed ulcers that form on the penis or entrance to the vagina.

132. Chemical Oxygen Demand (COD): The amount of chemical oxidation required to convert organic matter in water and waste water to CO_2.

133. Chemolithotropic Autotrophs: Microorganisms that oxidize reduced inorganic compounds to derive both energy and electrons; CO_2 is their carbon source. Also called chemolithoautotrophs.

134. Chemoorganotrophic Heterotrophs: Organisms that use organic compounds as sources of energy, hydrogen, electrons, and carbon for biosynthesis.

135. Chemostat: A continuous culture apparatus that feeds medium into the culture vessel at the same rate as medium containing microorganisms is removed; the medium in a chemostat contains one essential nutrient in a limiting quantity.

136. Chemotaxis: The pattern of microbial behaviour in which the microorganism moves toward chemical attractants and/or away from repellents.

137. Chemotherapeutic Agents: Compounds used in the treatment of disease that destroy pathogens or inhibit their growth at concentrations low enough to avoid doing undesirable damage to the host.

138. Chemotrophs: Organisms that obtain energy from the oxidation of chemical compounds.

139. Chickenpox (varicella): A highly contagious skin disease, usually affecting 2- to 7- year-old children; it is caused by the varicella-zoster virus, which is acquired by droplet inhalation into the respiratory system.

140. Chlamydiae: Members of the genus Chlamydia: gram-negative, coccoid cells that reproduce only within the cytoplasmic vesicles of host cells using a life cycle that alternates between elementary bodies and reticulate bodies.

141. Chlamydial Pneumonia: A penumonia caused by Chlamydia pneumoniae. Clinically, infections are mild and 50% of adults have antibodies to the chlamydiae.

142. Cholera: An acute infectious enteritis, endemic and epidemic in Asia, which periodically spreads to the Middle East, Africa, Southern Europe, and South America; caused by Vibrio cholerae.

143. Choleragen: The cholera toxin; an extremely potent protein molecule elaborated by strains of Vibrio cholerae in the small intestine after ingestion of feces-contaminated water or food. It acts on epithelial cells to cause hypersecretion of chloride and bicarbonate and an outpouring of large quantities of fluid from the mucosal surface.

144. Chromoblastomycosis: A chronic fungal skin infection, producing wartlike nodules that may ulcerate. It is caused by the black molds Phialophora verrucosa or Fonsecaea pedrosoi.

145. Cilia: Threadlike appendages extending from the surface of some protozoa that beat rhythmically to propel them; cilia are membrane-bound cylinders with a complex internal array of microtubules, usually in a 9 + 2 pattern.

146. Classical Complement Pathway: The antibody-dependent pathway of complement activation; it leads to the lysis of pathogens and stimulates phagocytosis and other host defenses.

147. Classification: The arrangement of organisms into groups based on mutual similarity or evolutionary relatedness.

148. Clone: A group of genetically identical cells or organisms derived by asexual reproduction from a single parent.

149. Coaggregation: The collection of a variety of bacteria on a surface such as a tooth surface because of cell-to-cell recognition of genetically distinct bacterial types. Many of these interactions appear to be mediated by a lectin on one bacterium that interacts with a complementary carbohydrate receptor on another bacterium.

150. Coagulase: An enzyme that induces blood clotting; it is characteristically produced by pathogenic staphylococci.

151. Coccidioidomycosis: A fungal disease caused by Coccidioides immitis that exists in dry, highly alkaline soils. Also known as valley fever, San Joaquin fever, or desert rheumatism.

152. Coccus: A roughly spherical bacterial cell.

153. Cold Sore: A lesion caused by the herpes simplex virus; usually occurs on the border of the lips or nares. Also known as a fever blister or herpes labialis.

154. Colicin: A plasmid-encoded protein that is produced by enteric bacteria and binds to specific receptors on the cell envelope of sensitive target bacteria, where it may cause lysis or attack specific intracellular sites such as ribosomes.

155. Coliform: A Gram-negative, non-sporing, facultative rod that ferments lactose with gas formation within 48 hours at 35°C.

156. Colonization: The establishment of a site of microbial reproduction on an inanimate surface or organism without necessarily resulting in tissue invasion or damage.

157. Colony: An assemblage of microorganisms growing on a solid surface such as the surface of an agar culture medium; the assemblage often is directly visible, but also may be seen only microscopically.

158. Colony Forming Units (CFU): The number of microorganisms that form colonies when cultured using spread plates or pour plates, an indication of the number of viable microorganisms in a sample.

159. Colorless Sulphur Bacteria: A diverse group of non-photosynthetic proteobacteria that can oxidize reduced sulfur compounds such as hydrogen sulfide. Many are lithotrophs and derive energy from sulfur oxidation. Some are unicellular, whereas others are filamentous gliding bacteria.

160. Combinatorial Biology: Introduction of genes from one microorganism into another microorganism to synthesize a new product or a modified product, especially in relation to antibiotic synthesis.

161. Cometabolism: The modification of a compound not used for growth by a microorganism, which occurs in the presence of another organic material that serves as a carbon and energy source.

162. Commensal: Living on or within another organism without injuring or benefiting the other organism.

163. Common Vehicle Transmission: The transmission of a pathogen to a host by means of an inanimate medium or vehicle.

164. Communicable Disease: A disease associated with a pathogen that can be transmitted from one host to another.

165. Competent: A bacterial cell that can take up free DNA fragments and incorporate them into its genome during transformation.

166. Competition: An interaction between two organisms attempting to use the same resource (nutrients, space, etc.).

167. Competitive Exclusion Principle: Two competing organisms overlap in resource use, which leads to the exclusion of one of the organisms.

168. Complex Medium: Culture medium that contains some ingredients of unknown chemical composition.

169. Complex Viruses: Viruses with capsids having a complex symmetry that is neither icosahedral nor helical.

170. Composting: The microbial processing of fresh organic matter under moist, aerobic conditions, resulting in the accumulation of a stable humified product, which is suitable for soil improvement and stimulation of plant growth.

171. Confocal Scanning Laser Microscope (CSLM): A light microscope in which monochromatic laser-derived light scans across the specimen at a specific level and illuminates one area at a time to form an image. Stray light from other parts of the specimen is blocked out to give an image with excellent contrast and resolution.

172. Congenital (neonatal) Herpes: A infection of a newbown caused by transmission of the herpesvirus during vaginal delivery.

173. Conjugation: The form of gene transfer and recombination in bacteria that requires direct cellto-cell contact 2. A complex form of sexual reproduction commonly employed by protozoa.

174. Conjugative Plasmid: A plasmid that carries the genes for sex pili and can transfer copies of itself to other bacteria during conjugation.

175. Conoid: A hollow cone of spirally coiled filaments in the anterior tip of certain apicomplexan protozoa.

176. Constitutive Mutant: A strain that produces as inducible enzyme continually, regardless of need, because of a mutation in either the operator or regulator gene.

177. Constructed Wetlands: Intentional creation of marshland plant communities and their associated microorganisms for environmental restoration or to purify water by the removal of bacteria, organic matter, and chemicals as the water passes through the aquatic plant communities.

178. Consumer: An organism that feeds directly on living or dead animals, by ingestion or by phagocytosis.

179. Contact Transmission: Transmission of the pathogen by contact of the source or reservoir of the pathogen with the host.

180. Continuous Culture System: A culture system with constant environmental conditions maintained through continual provision of nutrients and removal of wastes.

181. Convalescent Carrier: An individual who has recovered from an infectious disease but continues to harbor large numbers of the pathogen.

182. Cooperation: A positive but not obiligatory interaction between two different organisms. Also called protocooperation.

183. Cortex: The layer of a bacterial endospore that is thought to be particularly important in conferring heat resistance on the endospore.

184. Cryptococcosis: An infection caused by the basidiomycete. Cryptococcus neoformans, which may involve the skin, lungs, brain, or meninges.

185. Cryptosporidiosis: Infection with protozoa of the genus Crypto-sporidium. The most common symptoms are prolonged diarrhea, weight loss, fever, and abdominal pain.

186. Cutaneous Diphtheria: A skin disease caused by Corynebacterium diphtheriae that infects wound or skin lesions, causing a slow-healing ulceration.

187. Cyanobacteria: A large group of bacteria that carry out oxygenic photosynthesis using a system like that present in photosynthetic eucaryotes.

188. Cyst: A general term used for a specialized microbial cell enclosed in a wall. Cysts are formed by protozoa and a few bacteria. They may be dormant, resistant structures formed in response to adverse conditions or reproductive cysts that are a normal stage in the life cycle.

189. Cytopathic Effect: The observable change that occurs in cells as a result of viral replication. Examples include ballooning, binding together, clustering, or ever death of the cultured cells.

190. Cytoplasmic Matrix: The protoplasm of a cell that lies within the plasma membrane and outside any other organelles. In bacteria it is the substance between the cell membrane and the nucleoid.

191. Cytotoxin. A toxin or antibody that has a specific toxic action upto cells; cytotoxins are named according to the cell for which they are specific (e.g., nephrotoxin).

192. Dane Particle: A 42 nm spherical particle that is one of three that are seen in hepatitis B virus infections. The Dane particle is the complete virion.

193. Dark-Field Microscopy: Microscopy in which the specimen is brightly illuminated while the background is dark.

194. Death Phase: The decrease in viable microorganisms that occurs after the completion of growth in a batch culture.

195. Decimal Reduction Time (D or D value): The time required to kill 90% of the microorganisms or spores in a sample at a specified temperature.

196. Decomposer: An organism that breaks down complex materials into simpler ones, including the release of simple inorganic products. Often a decomposersuch as an insect or earthworm physically reduces the size of substrate particles.

197. Defensin: Specific peptides produced by neutrophils that permeabilize the outer and inner membranes of certain microorganisms, thus killing them.

198. Defined Medium: Culture medium made with components of known composition.

199. Delta-proteobacteria: One of the five subgroups of proteobacteria. Chemoorganotrophic bacteria that usually are either predators on other bacteria or anaerobes that generate sulfide from sulfate and sulfite.

200. Dendrogram: A treelike diagram that is used to graphically summarize mutual similarities and relationships between organisms.

201. Denitrification: The reduction of nitrate to gaseous products, primarily nitrogen gas, during anaerobic respiration.

202. Dental Plaque: A thin film on the surface of teeth consisting of bacteria embedded in a matrix of bacterial polysaccharides, salivary glycoproteins, and other substances.

203. Deoxyribonucleic Acid (DNA): The nucleic acid that constitutes the genetic material of all cellular organisms. It is a polynucleotide composed of deoxyribonucleotides connected by phosphodiester bonds.

204. Dermatomycosis: A fungal infection of the skin; the term is a general term that comprises the various forms of tinea, and it is sometimes used to specifically refer to athelete's foot (tinea pedis).

205. Desert Crust: A crust formed by microbial binding of sand grains in the surface zone of desert soil; crust formation primarily involves cyanobacteria.

206. Detergent: An organic molecule, other than a soap, that serves as a wetting agent and emulsifier; it is normally used as cleanser. But some may be used as antimicrobial agents.

207. Deuteromycetes: In some classification systems, the deuteromycetes or Fungi Imperfecti are a class of fungi. These organisms either lack a sexual stage or it has not yet been discovered.

208. Diauxic Growth: A biphasic growth pattern or response in which a microorganism, when exposed to two nutrients, initially uses one of them for growth and then alters its metabolism to make use of the second.

209. Differential Interference Contrast (DIC) Microscope. A light microscope that employs two beams of plane polarized light. The beams are combined after passing through the specimen and their interference is used to create the image.

210. Differential Media: Culture media that distinguish between groups of microorganisms based on differences in their growth and metabolic products.

211. Differential Staining Procedures: Staining procedures that divide bacteria into separate groups based on staining properties.

212. Diffusely Adhering E. coli (DAEC): DAEC strains of E. coli adhere over the entire surface of epithelial cells and usually cause diarrheal disease in immunologically naive and malnourished children.

213. Dikaryotic Stage: In fungi, having pairs of nuclei within cells or compartments. Each cell contains two separate haploid nuclei, one from each parent.

214. Dinoflagellate: An algal protist characterized by two flagella used in swimming in a spinning pattern. Many are bioluminescentand an important part of marine phytoplankton, some also are importantmarine pathogens.

215. Diphtheria: An acute, highly contagious childhood disease that generally affects the membranes of the throat and less frequently the nose. It is caused by Corynebacterium diphtheriae.

216. Dipicolinic Acid: A substance present at high concentrations in the bacterial endspore. It is thought to contribute to the endospore's heat resistance.

217. Diplococcus: A pair of cocci.

218. Directed or Adaptive Mutation: A mutation that seems to be chosen so the organism can better adapt to its surroundings.

219. Disinfectant: An agent, usually chemical, that disinfects; normally, it is employed only with inanimate objects.

220. Disinfection: The killing, inhibition, or removal of microorganisms that may cause disease. It usually refers to the treatment of inanimate objects with chemicals.

221. Disinfection By-products (DBPs): Chlorinated organic compounds such as trihalomethanes formed during chlorine use for water disinfection. Many are carcinogens.

222. Dissimilatory Nitrate Reduction: The process in which some bacteria use nitrate as the electron acceptor at the end of their electron transport chain to produce ATP. The nitrate is reduced to nitrite or nitrogen gas.

223. Dissimilatory Reduction: The use of a substance as an electron acceptor in energy generation. The acceptor (e.g., sulfate or nitrate) is reduced but not incorporated into organic matter during biosynthetic processes.

224. DNA Vaccine: A vaccine that contains DNA which encodes antigenic proteins. It is injected directly into the muscle; the DNA is taken up by the muscle cells and encoded protein antigens are synthesized. This produces both humoral and cell-mediated responses.

225. Eclipse Period: The initial part of the latent period in which infected host bacteria do not contain any complete virions.

226. Effacing Lesion: The type of lesion caused by enteropathogenic strains of E. coli (EPEC) when the bacteria destroy the brush border of intestinal epithelial cells. The term AE (attaching-effacing) E. coli is now used to designate true EPEC strains that are an important cause of diarrhea in children from developing countries and in traveler's diarrhoea.

227. Ehrlichiosis: A tick-borne (Dermacentor andersoni, Amblyomma americanum) rickettsial disease caused by Ehrlichia chaffeensis. Once inside leukocytes, a nonspecific illness develops that resembles Rocky Mountain spotted fever.

228. Endogenous Infection: An infection by a member of an individual's own normal body microbiota.

229. Endosymbiont: An organism that lives within the body of another organism in a symbiotic association.

230. Endosymbiosis: A type of symbiosis in which one organism is found within another organism.

231. Endosymbiotic Theory or Hypothesis: The theory that eucaryotic organelles such as mitochondria and chloroplasts arose when bacteria established an endosymbiotic relationship with the eucaryotic ancestor and then evolved into organelles.

232. Enteric Bacteria (enterobacteria): Members of the family Enterobacteriaceae (Gram-negative, peritrichous or nonmotile, facultatively anaerobic, straight rods with simple nutritional requirements); also used for bacteria that live in the intestinal tract.

233. Enterohemorrhagic E. coli (EHEC): EHEC strains of E. coli (O157:H7) produce several cytotoxins that provoke fluids secretion in traveller's diarrhea; however, their mode of action is unknown.

234. Enterionvasive E. coli (EIEC): EIEC strains of E. coli cause traveller's diarrhoea by penetrating and binding to the intestinal epithelial cells, EIEC may also produce a cytotoxin and enterotoxin.

235. Enteropathogenic E. coli (EPEC): EPEC strains of E. coli attach to the brush border of intestinal epithelial cells and cause a specific type of cell damage called effacing lesions that lead to traveller's diarrhea.

236. Enterotoxigenic E. coli (ETEC): ETEC strains of E. coli produce two plasmid-encoded enterotoxins (which are responsible for traveller's diarrhea) and the distinguished by their heat stability: heat-stable enterotoxin (ST) and heat-labile enterotoxin (LT).

237. Epidemic (louse-borne) Typhus: A disease caused by Rickettsia prowazekii that is transmitted from person to person by the body louse.

238. Epsilon-proteobacteria: One of the five subgroups of proteo-bacteria, each with distinctive 16S rRNA sequences. Slender Gram-negative rods, some of which are medically important (Campylobacter and Helicobacter).

239. Ergot: The dried sclerotium of Claviceps purpurea. Also, an ascomycete that parasitizes rye and other higher plants causing the disease called ergotism.

240. Ergotism: The disease or toxic condition caused by eating grain infected with ergot; it is often accompanied by gangrene, psychotic delusions, nervous spasms, abortion, and convulsions in humans and in animals.

241. Eucarya: The domain that contains organisms composed of eucaryotic cells with primarily glycerol fatty acyl diesters in their membranes and eucaryotic rRNA.

242. Excystation: The escape of one or more cells or organisms from a cyst.

243. Exergonic reaction: A reaction that spontaneously goes to completion as written; the standard free energy change is negative, and the equilibrium constant is greater than one.

244. Exogenote: The piece of donor DNA that enters a bacterial cell during gene exchange and recombination.

245. Exotoxin: A heat-labile, toxic protein produced by a bacterium as a result of its normal metabolism or because of the acquisition of a plasmid or prophage. It is usually released into the bacterium's surroundings.

246. Exponential Phase: The phase of the growth curve during which the microbial population is growing at a constant and maximum rate, dividing and doubling at regular intervals.

247. Extracutaneous Sporotrichosis: An infection by the fungus Sporothrix schenckii that spreads throughout the body.

248. Extreme Barophilic Bacteria: Bacteria that require a high-pressure environment to function.

249. Extreme Environment: An environment in which physical factors such as temperature, pH, salinity, and pressure are outside of the normal range for growth of most microorganisms; these conditions allow unique organisms to survive and function.

250. Extremophiles: Microorganisms that grow under harsh or extreme environmental conditions such as very high temperatures or low pHs.

251. Extrinsic Factor: An environmental factor such as temperature that influences microbial growth in food.

252. Facultative Anaerobes: Microorganisms that do not require oxygen for growth, but do grow better in its presence.

253. Fecal Coliform: Coliforms whose normal habitat is the intestinal tract and that can grow at 44.5°C.

254. Fecal Enterococci: Enterococci found in the intestine of humans and other warm-blooded animals. They are used as indicators of the fecal pollution of water.

255. Fimbria (fimbriae): A fine, hairlike protein appendage on some gram-negative bacteria that helps attach them to surfaces.

256. Flagellin: The protein used to construct the filament of a bacterial flagellum.

257. Flagellum (flagella): A thin, threadlike appendage on many prokaryotic and eukaryotic cells that is responsible for their motility.

258. Fluorescence Microscope: A microscope that exposes a specimen to light of a specific wavelength and then forms an image from the fluorescent light produced. Usually the specimen is stained with a fluorescent dye or fluorochrome.

259. Fomite (fomites): An object that is not in itself harmful but is able to harbor and transmit pathogenic organisms. Also called fomes.

260. Food-borne Infection: Gastrointestinal illness caused by ingestion of microorganisms, followed by their growth within the host. Symptoms arise from tissue invasion and/or toxin production.

261. Food Web: A network of many interlinked food chains, encompassing primary producers, consumers, decomposers and detritivores.

262. Gamma-proteobacteria: One of the five sub-groups of proteobacteria, each with distinctive 16S rRNA sequences. This is the largest subgroup and is very diverse physiologically; many important genera are facultatively anaerobic chemoorganotrophs.

263. Gas Gangrene: A type of gangrene that arises from dirty, lacerated wounds infected by anaerobic bacteria, especially species of Clostridium. As the bacteria grow, they release toxins and ferment carbohydrates to produce carbon dioxide and hydrogen gas.

264. Gastroenteritis: An acute inflammation of the lining of the stomach and intestines, characterized by anorexia, nausea, diarrhea, abdominal pain, and weakness. It has various causes including food poisoning due to such organisms as E. coli, S. aureus, Campylobacter (campylobacteriosis) and Salmonella species; consumption of irritating food or drink; or psychological factors such as anger, stress, and fear. Also called enterogastritis.

265. Gas Vacuole: A gas-filled vacuole found in cyanobacteria and some other aquatic bacteria that provides flotation. It is composed of gas vesicles, which are made of protein.

266. Generalized Transduction: The transfer of any part of a bacterial genome when the DNA fragment is packaged within a phage capsid by mistake.

267. General Recombination: Recombination involving a reciprocal exchange of a pair of homologous DNA sequences; it can occur any place on the chromosome.

268. Generation Time: The time required for a microbial population to double in number.

269. Genetic Engineering: The deliberate modification of an organism's genetic information by directly changing its nucleic acid genome.

270. Genital Herpes: A sexually transmitted disease caused by the herpes simplex virus type 2.

271. Germicide: An agent that kills pathogens and many nonpathogens but not necessarily bacterial endospores.

272. Giardiasis: A common intestinal disease caused by the parasitic protozoan Giardia lamblia.

273. Glycocalyx: A network of polysaccharides extending from the surface of bacteria and other cells.

274. Gnotobiotic: Animals that are germfree (microorganisms free) or live in association with one or more known microorganisms.

275. Gonococci: Bacteria of the species Neisseria gonorrhoeae—the organism causing gonorrhea.

276. Gonorrhea: An acute infectious sexually transmitted disease of the mucous membranes of the genitourinary tract, eye, rectum, and throat. It is caused by Neisseria gonorrhoeae.

277. Gram Stain: A differential staining procedure that divides bacteria into Gram-positive and Gramnegative groups based on their ability to retain crystal violet when decolorized with an organic solvent such as ethanol.

278. Greenhouse Gases: Gases released from the Earth's surface through chemical and biological processes that interact with the chemicals in the stratosphere to decrease the release of radiation from the Earth. It is believed that this leads to global warming.

279. Guillain-Barré Syndrome: A relatively rare disease affecting the peripheral nervous system, especially the spinal nerves, but also the cranial nerves. The cause is unknown, but it most often occurs after an influenza infection or flu vaccination. Also called French Polio.

280. Halophile: A microorganism that requires high levels of sodium chloride for growth.

281. Harborage Transmission: The mode of transmission in which an infectious organism does not undergo morphological or physiological changes within the vector.

282. Healthy Carrier: An individual who harbors a pathogen, but is not ill.

283. Hemolysis: The disruption of red blood cells and release of their hemoglobin. There are several types of hemolysis when bacteria such as streptococci and staphylococci, grow on blood agar. In α-hemolysis, a narrow greenish zone of incomplete hemolysis forms around the colony. A clear zone of complete hemolysis without any obvious colour change is formed during β-hemolysis.

284. Hemolytic Uremic Syndrome: A kidney disease characterized by blood in the urine and often by kidney failure. It is caused by enterohemorrhagic strains of Escherichia coli O157 : H7 that produce a Shiga-like toxin, which attacks the kidneys.

285. Hepatitis A. (formerly infectious hepatitis): A type of hepatitis that is transmitted by fecal - oral contamination; it primarily affects children and young adults, especially in environments where there is poor sanitation and overcrowding. It is caused by the hepatitis A virus, a singlestranded RNA virus.

286. Hepatitis B. (formely serum hepatitis): This form of hepatitis is caused by a double-stranded DNA virus (HBV) formerly called the "DNA particle". The virus is transmitted by body fluids.

287. Hepatitis C: About 90% of all cases of viral hepatitis can be traced to either HAV or HBV. The remaining 10% is believed to be caused by one and possibly several other types of viruses. At least one of these is hepatitis C (formerly non-A, non-B).

288. Hepatitis D (formerly delta hepatitis): The liver diseases caused by the hepatitis D virus in those individuals already infected with the hepatitis B virus.

289. Hepatitis E (formerly enteric-transmitted NANB hepatitis): The liver disease caused by the hepatitis E virus. Usually, a subclinical, acute infection results, however, there is a high mortality in women in their last trimester of pregnancy.

290. Heterolactic Fermenters: Microorganisms that ferment sugars to form lactate and also other products such as ethanol and CO_2.

291. Heterotroph: An organism that uses reduced, preformed organic molecules as its principal carbonsource.

292. Heterotrophic Nitrification: Nitrification carried out by chemohetero-trophic microorganisms.

293. Hfr strain: A bacterial strain that denotes its genes with high frequency to a recipient cell during conjugation because the F factor is integrated into the bacterial chromosome.

294. High Oxygen Diffusion Environment: A microbial environment in close contact with air and through which oxygen can move at a rapid rate (in comparison wtih the slow diffusion rate of oxygen through water).

295. Holdfast: A structure produced by some bacteria and algae that attaches them to a solid object.

296. Holozoic Nutrition: In this type of nutrition, nutrients (such as bacteria) are acquired by phagocytosis and the subsequent formation of a food vacuole or phagosome.

297. Homolactic Fermenters: Organisms that ferment sugars almost completely to lactic acid.

298. Host: The body of an organism that harbors another organism. It can be viewed as a microenvironment that shelters and supports the growth and multiplication of a parasitic organism.

299. Host Restriction: The degradation of foreign genetic material by nucleases after the genetic material enters a host cell.

300. Human Immunodeficiency Virus (HIV): A lentivirus of the family, Retroviridae that is associated with the onset of AIDS.

301. Hypermutation: A rapid production of multiple mutations in a gene or genes through the activation of special mutator genes. The process may be deliberately used to maximize the possibility of creating desirable mutants.

302. Hyperthermophile: A bacterium that has its growth optimum between 80°C and about 113°C. Hyperthermophiles usually do not grow well below 55°C.

303. Hypha (hyphae): The unit of structure of most fungi and some bacteria; a tubular filament.

304. Identification: The process of determining that a particular, isolate or organism belongs to a recognized taxon.

305. Immobilization: The incorporation of a simple, soluble substance into the body of an organism, making it unavailable for use by other organisms.

306. Inclusion Bodies: Granules of organic or inorganic material lying in the cytoplasmic matrix of bacteria.

307. Inclusion Conjunctivitis: An infectitious disease that occurs worldwide. It is caused by Chlamydia trachomatis that infects the eye and causes inflammation and the occurrence of large inclusion bodies.

308. Incubation Period: The period after pathogen entry into a host and before signs and symptoms appear.

309. Incubatory Carrier: An individual who is incubating a pathogen but is not yet ill.

310. Indicator Organism: An organism whose presence indicates the condition of a substance or environment, for example, the potential presence of pathogens. Coliforms are used as indicators of fecal pollution.

311. Infection: The invasion of a host by a microorganism with subsequent establishment and multiplication of the agent. An infection may or may not lead to overt disease.

312. Infection Thread: A tubular structure formed during the infection of a root by nitrogen-fixing bacteria. The bacteria enter the root by way of the infection thread and stimulate the formation of the root nodule.

313. Infectious Disease Cycle (Chain of Infection): The chain or cycle of events that describes how an infectious organism grows, reproduces, and is disseminated.

314. Infectious Dose 50 (ID50): Refers to the dose or number of organisms that will infect 50% of an experimental group of hosts within a specified time period.

315. Infectivity: Infectiousness; the state or quality of being infectious or communicable.

316. Integration: The incorporation of one DNA segment into a second DNA molecule to form a new hybrid DNA. Integration occurs during such processes as genetic recombination, episome incorporation into host DNA, and prophage insertion into the bacterial chromosome.

317. Integrins: A large family of α/β heterodimers. Integrins are cellular adhesion receptors that mediate cell-cell and cell-substratum interactions. Integrins usually recognize linear amino acid sequences on protein ligands.

318. Integron: A genetic element with an attachment site for site-specific recombination and an integrase gene. It can capture genes and gene cassettes.

319. Intercalating Agents: Molecules that can be inserted between the stacked bases of a DNA double helix, thereby distorting the DNA and including insertion and deletion mutations.

320. Interferon (IFN): A glycoprotein that has nonspecific antiviral activity by stimulating cells to produce antiviral proteins, which inhibit the synthesis of viral RNA and proteins. Interferonsalso regulate the growth, differentiation, and/or function of a variety of immune system cells. Their production may be stimulated by virus infections, intracellular pathogens (chlamydiae and rickettsias), protozoan parasites, endotoxins, and other agents.

321. Interleukin: A glycoprotein produced by macrophages and T cells that regulates growth and differentiation, particularly of lymphocytes. Interleukins promote cellular and humoral immune responses.

322. Intermediate Filaments: Small protein filaments about 8 to 10 nm in diameter, in the cytoplasmic matrix of eucaryotic cells that are important in cell structure.

323. Interspecies Hydrogen Transfer: The linkage of hydrogen production from organic matter by anaerobic heterotrophic microorganisms to the use of hydrogen by other anaerobes in the reduction of carbon dioxide to methane. This avoids possible hydrogen toxicity.

324. Intertriginous Candidiasis: A skin infection caused by Candida species. Involves those areas of the body, usually opposed skin surfaces, that are warm and moist (axillae, groin, skin folds).

325. Intoxication: A disease that results from the entrance of a specific toxin into the body of a host. The toxin can induce the disease in the absence of the toxin producing organisms.

326. Intrinsic Factors: Food-related factors such as moisture, pH, and available nutrients that influence microbial growth.

327. Invasiveness: The ability of a microorganism to enter a host, grow and reproduce within the host, and spread throughout its body.

328. Kirby-Bauer Method: A disk diffusion test to determine the susceptibility of a microorganism to chemotherapeutic agents.

329. Koch's Postulates: A set of rules for proving that microorganism causes a particular disease.

330. Lactic Acid Fermentation: A fermentation that produces lactic acid as the sole or primary product.

331. Lager: Pertaining to the process of aging beers to allow flavor development.

332. Lag Phase: A period following the introduction of microorganisms into fresh culture medium when there is no increase in cell numbers or mass during batch culture.

333. Latent Period: The initial phase in the one-step growth experiment in which no phages are released.

334. Lectin Complement Pathway: The lectin pathway for complement activation is triggered by the binding of a serum lectin (mannan-binding lectin; MBL) to mannose-containing proteins or to carbohydrates on viruses or bacteria.

335. Leishmanias: Zooflagellates, members of the genus Leishmania, that cause the disease leishmaniasis.

336. Leishmaniasis: The disease caused by the protozoa called leishmanias.

337. Lepromatous (progressive) Leprosy. A relentless, progressive form of leprosy in which large numbers of Mycobacterium lepae develop in skin cells, killing the skin cells and resulting in the loss of features. Disfiguring nodules from all over the body.

338. Leprosy or Hansen's Disease: A severe disfiguring skin disease caused by Mycobacteriumleprae.

339. Lethal Dose 50 (LD50): Refers to the dose or number of organisms that will kill 50% of an experimental group of hosts within a specified time period.

340. Leukemia: A progressive, malignant disease of blood-forming organs, marked by distorted proliferation anddevelopment of leukocytes and their precursors in the blood and bone marrow. Certain leukemias are caused by viruses (HTLV-1, HTLV-2).

341. Leukocidin: A microbial toxin that can damage or kill leukocytes.

342. Lichen: An organism composed of a fungus and either green algae or cyanobacteria in a symbiotic association.

343. Liebig's Law of the Minimum: Living organisms and populations will grow until lack of a resource begins to limit further growth.

344. Lipopolysaccharide (LPSs): A molecule containing both lipid and polysaccharide, which is important in the outer membrane of the Gram-negative cell wall.

345. Listeriosis: A sporadic disease of animals and humans, particularly those who are immunocompromised or pregnant, caused by the bacterium Listeria monocytogenes.

346. Lithotroph: An organism that uses reduced inorganic compounds as its electron source.

347. Low Oxygen Diffusion Environment: An aquatic environment in which microorganisms are surrounded by deep water layers that limit oxygen-diffusion to the cell surface. In contrast, microorganisms in thin water films have good oxygen transfer from air to the cell surface.

348. LPS-Binding Protein: A special plasma protein that binds bacterial lipopolysaccharides and then attaches to receptors on monocytes, macrophages, and other cells. This triggers the release of IL-1 and other cytokines that stimulate the development of fever and additional endotoxin effects.

349. Lymphogranuloma Venereum (LGV): A sexually transmitted disease caused by Chalmydia trachomatis serotypes L1 – L3, which affect the lymph organs in the genital area.

350. Lysogens: Bacteria that are carrying a viral prophage and can produce bacteriophages under the proper conditions.

351. Lysogeny: The state in which a phage genome remains within the bacterial cell after infection and reproduces along with it rather than taking control of the host and destroying it.

352. Lysosome: A spherical membranous eucaryotic organelle that contains hydrolytic enzymes and is responsible for the intracellular digestion of substances.

353. Macrolide Antibiotic: An antibiotic containing a macrolide ring, a large lactone ring with multiple keto and hydroxyl groups, linked to one or more sugars.

354. Macromolecule Vaccine: A vaccine made of specific, purified macromolecules derived from pathogenic microorganisms.

355. Macronucleus: The larger of the two nuclei in ciliate protozoa. It is normally popyploid and directs the routine activities of the cell.

356. Macrophage: The name for a large mononuclear phagocytic cell, present in blood, lymph and other tissues. Macrophages are derived from monocytes. They phagocytose and destroy pathogens; some macrophages also activate B cells and T cells.

357. Maduromycosis: A subcutaneous fungal infection caused by Madurella mycetoma; also termed an eumycotic mycetoma.

358. Madurose: The sugar derivative 3-O-methyl-D-galactose, which is characteristic of several actinomycete genera that are collectively called maduromycetes.

359. Magnetosomes: Magnetite particles in magnetotactic bacteria that are tiny magnets and allow the bacteria to orient themselves in magnetic fields.

360. Malaria: A serious infectious illness caused by the parasitic protozoan Plasmodium. Malaria is characterized by bouts of high chills and fever that occur at regular intervals.

361. Mash: The soluble materials released from germinated grains and prepared as a microbial growth medium.

362. Mean Growth Rate Constant (k): The rate of microbial population growth expressed in terms of the number of generations per unit time.

363. Meiosis: The sexual process in which a diploid cell divides and forms two haploid cells.

364. Melting Temperature (Tm): The temperature at which double-standard DNA separates into individual strands; it is dependent on the G + C content of the DNA and is used to compare genetic material in microbial taxonomy.

365. Membrane Filter Technique: The use of a thin porous filter made from cellulose acetate or some other polymer to collect microorganisms from water, air and food.

366. Meningitis: A condition that refers to inflammation of the brain or spinal cord meninges (membranes). The disease can be divided into bacterial (septic) meningitis and aseptic meningitis syndrome (caused by nonbacterial sources).

367. Mesophile: A microorganism with a growth optimum around 20 to 45°C, a minimum of 15 to 20°C and a maximum about 45°C or lower.

368. Metachromatic Granules: Granules of polyphosphate in the cytoplasm of some bacteria that appear a different colour when stained with a blue basic dye. They are storage reservoirs for phosphate. Sometimes called volutin granules.

369. Methanogens: Strictly anaerobic archaeons that derive energy by converting CO_2, H_2, formate, acetate, and other compounds to either methane or methane and CO_2.

370. Methylotroph: A bacterium that uses reduced one-carbon compounds such as methane and methanol as its sole source of carbon and energy.

371. Microaerophile: A microorganism that requires low levels of oxygen for growth, around 2 to 10%, but is damaged by normal atmospheric oxygen levels.

372. Microbial Ecology: The study of microorganisms in their natural environments, with a major emphasis on physical conditions, processes, and interactions that occur on the scale of individual microbial cells.

373. Microbial Loop: The mineralization of organic matter synthesized by photosynthetic phytoplankton through the activity of microorganisms such as bacteria and protozoa. This process "loops" minerals and carbon dioxide back for reuse by the primary producers and makes the organic matter unavailable to higher consumers.

374. Microbial Mat: A firm structure of layered microorganisms with complementary physiological activities that can develop on surfaces in aquatic environments.

375. Microbiology: The study of organisms that are usually too small to be seen with the naked eye. Special techniques are required to isolate and grow them.

376. Microbivory: The use of microorganisms as a food source by organisms that can ingest or phagocytose them.

377. Microenvironment: The immediate environment surrounding a microbial cell or other structure, such as a root.

378. Microorganism: An organism that is too small to be seen clearly with the naked eye.

379. Miliary Tuberculosis: An acute form of tuberculosis in which small tubercles are formed in a number of organs of the body because of disemination of M. tuberculosis throughout the body by the bloodstream. Also known as reactivation tuberculosis.

380. Mineralization: The release of inorganic nutrients from organic matter during microbial growth and metabolism.

381. Minimal Inhibitory Concentration (MIC): The lowest concentration of a drug that will prevent the growth of a particular microorganism.

382. Minimal Lethal Concentration (MLC): The lowest concentration of a drug that will kill a particular microorganism.

383. Mitochondrion: The eucaryotic organelle that is the site of electron transport, oxidative phosphorylation, and pathways such as the Krebs cycle; it provides most of a nonphotosynthetic cell's energy under aerobic conditions. It is constructed of an outer membrane and an inner membrane, which contains the electron transport chain.

384. Mitosis: A process that takes place in the nucleus of a eucaryotic cell and results in the formation of two new nuclei, each with the same number of chromosomes as the parent.

385. Mixed Acid Fermentation: A type of fermentation carried out by members of the family Enterobacteriaceae in which ethanol and a complex mixture of organic acids are produced.

386. Mixotrophic: Refers to microorganisms that combine autotrophic and heterotrophic metabolic processes (they use inorganic electron sources and organic carbon sources).

387. Modified Atmosphere Packaging (MAP): Addition of gases such as nitrogen and carbon dioxide to packaged foods in order to inhibit the growth of spoilage organisms.

388. Mold: Any of a large group of fungi that cause mold or moldiness and that exist as multicellular filamentous colonies; also the deposit or growth caused by such fungi. Molds typically do not produce macroscopic fruiting bodies.

389. Most Probable Number (MPN): The statistical estimation of the probable population in a liquid by diluting and determining end points for microbial growth.

390. Mucociliary Blanket: The layer of cilia and mucus that lines certain portions of the respiratory system; it traps microorganisms up to 10 μm in diameter and then transports them by ciliary action away from the lungs.

391. Mucociliary Escalator: The mechanism by which respiratory ciliated cells move material and microorganisms, trapped in mucus, out of the pharynx, where it is spit out or swallowed.

392. Multi-drug-resistant Strains of Tuberculosis (MDR-TB): A multi-drug-resistant strain is defined as Mycobacterium tuberculosis resistant to isoniazid and rifampin, with or without resistance to other drugs.

393. Mutation: A permanent, heritable change in the genetic material.

394. Mutualist: An organism associated with another in an obligatory relationship that is beneficial to both.

395. Mycelium: A mass of branching hyphae found in fungi and some bacteria.

396. Mycolic Acids: Complex 60 to 90 carbon fatty acids with a hydroxyl on the β-carbon and an aliphatic chain on the α-carbon, found in the cell walls of mycobacteria.

397. Mycoplasma: Bacteria that are members of the class Mollicutes and order Mycoplasmatales; they lack cell walls and cannot synthesize peptidoglycan precursors; most require sterols for growth; they are the smallest organisms capable of independent reproduction.

398. Mycoplasmal Pneumonia: A type of pneumonia caused by Mycoplasma pneumoniae. Spread involves airborne droplets and close contact.

399. Mycorrhizosphere: The region around ectomycorrhizal mantles and hyphae in which nutrients released from the fungus increase the microbial population and its activities.

400. Mycotoxicology: The study of fungal toxins and their effects on various organisms.

401. Myxobacteria: A group of Gram-negative, aerobic soil bacteria characterized by gliding motility, a complex life cycle with the production of fruiting bodies, and the formation of myxospores.

402. Myxospores: Special dormant spores formed by the myxobacteria.

403. Narrow-spectrum Drugs: Chemotherapeutic agents that are effective only against a limited variety of microorganisms.

404. Natural Classification: A classification system that arranges organisms into groups whose members share many characteristics and reflect as much as possible the biological nature of organisms.

405. Necrotizing Fasciitis: A disease that results from a severe invasive group. A streptococcus infection. Necrotizing fasciitis is an infection of the subcutanious soft tissues, particularly of fibrous tissue, and is most common on the extremities. It begins with skin reddening, swelling, pain and cellulitis and proceeds to skin breakdown and gangrene after 3 to 5 days.

406. Negative Staining: A staining procedure in which a dye is used to make the background dark while the specimen is unstained.

407. Neurotoxin: A toxin that is poisonous to or destroys nerve tissue; especially the toxins secreted by C. tetani, Corynebacterium diphtheriae, and Shigella dysrenteriae.

408. Neustonic: The microorganisms that live at the atmospheric interface of a water body.

409. Neutrophile: Microorgansims that grow best at a neutral pH range between pH 5.5 and 8.0.

410. Niche: The function of an organism in a complex system, including place of the organism, the resources used in a given location, and the time of use.

411. Nitrifying Bacteria: Chemolithotrophic, Gram-negative bacteria that are members of the family Nitrobacteriaceae and convert ammonia to nitrate and nitrite to nitrate.

412. Nitrogen Fixation: The metabolic process in which atmospheric molecular nitrogen is reduced to ammonia; carried out by cyanobacteria, Rhizobium and other nitrogen-fixing procaryotes.

413. Nitrogen Oxygen Demand (NOD). The demand for oxygen is sewage treatment, caused by nitrifying microorganisms.

414. Nocardioforms. Bacteria that resemble members of the genus Nocardia; they develop a substrate mycelium that readily breaks up into rods and coccoid elements (a quality sometimes called fugacity).

415. Nomenclature: The branch of taxonomy concerned with the assignment of names to taxonomic groups in agreement with published rules.

416. Nondiscrete Microorganism: A microorganism, best exemplified by a filamentous fungus, that does not have a defined and predictable cell structure or distinct edges and boundaries. The organism can be defined in terms of the cell structure and its cytoplasmic contents.

417. Normal Microbiota (also indigenous microbial population, microflora, microbial flora): The microorganisms normally associated with a particular tissue or structure.

418. Nucleoid: An irregularly shaped region in the procaryotic cell that contains its genetic material.

419. Nucleolus: The organelle, located within the eucaryotic nucleus and not bounded by a membrane, that is the location of ribosomal RNA synthesis and the assembly of ribosomal subunits.

420. Numerical Aperture: The property of a microscope lens that determines how much light can enter and how great a resolution the lens can provide.

421. Nutrient: A substance that supports growth and reproduction.

422. Nystatin: A polyene antibiotic from *Streptomyces noursei* that is used in the treatment of Candida infections of the skin, vagina and alimentary tract.

423. O Antigen: A polysaccharide antigen extending from the outer membrane of some gram-negative bacterial cell walls; it is part of the lipopolysaccharide.

424. Obligate Anaerobes: Microorganisms that cannot tolerate the presence of oxygen and die when exposed to it.

425. One-step Growth Experiment: An experiment used to study the reproduction of lytic phages in which one round of phage reproduction occurs and ends with the lysis of the host bacterial population.

426. Open Reading Frame (ORF): A reading frame sequence not interrupted by a stop codon; it is usually determined by nucleic acid sequencing studies.

427. Opportunistic Microorganism or Pathogen: A microorganism that is usually free-living or a part of the host's normal microbiota, but which may become pathogenic under certain circumstances, such as when the immune system is compromised.

428. Opsonization: The action of opsonins in making bacteria and other cells more readily phagocytosed. Antibodies, complement (especially C3b) and fibronectin are potent opsonins.

429. Optical Tweezer: The use of a focused laser beam to drag and isolate a specific microorganism from a complex microbial mixture.

430. Organotrophs: Organisms that use reduced organic compounds as their electron source.

431. Osmophilic Microorganisms: Microorgnisms that grow best in or on media of high solute concentration.

432. Osmotolerant: Organisms that grow over a fairly wide range of water activity or solute concentration.

433. Outer Membrane: A special membrane located outside the peptidoglycan layer in the cell walls of Gram-negative bacteria.

434. Oxidative Burst: The generation of reactive oxygen species, primarily superoxide anion ($-O2$) and hydrogen peroxide ($H2O_2$) by a plant or an animal, in response to challenge by a potential bacterial, fungal, or viral pathogen.

435. Oxygenic Photosynthesis: Photosynthesis that oxidizes water to form oxygen ; the form of photosynthesis characteristic of algae and cyanobacteria.

436. Parasite: An organism that lives on or within another organism (the host) and benefits from the association while harming its host. Often the parasite obtains nutrients from the host.

437. Parasitism: A type of symbiosis in which one organism benefits from the other and the host is usually harmed.

438. Parfocal: A microscope that retains proper focus when the objectives are changed.

439. Pasteur Effect: The decrease in the rate of sugar catobolism and change to aerobic respiration that occurs when microorganisms are switched from anaerobic to aerobic conditions.

440. Pasteurization: The process of heating milk and other liquids to destroy microorgnisms that can cause spoilage or disease.

441. Pathogen: Any virus, bacterium, or other agent that causes disease.

442. Pathogen-Associated Molecular Pattern (PAMP): Conserved molecular structures that occur in patterns on microbial surfaces. The structures and their patterns are unique to particular microorganisms and invariant among members of a given microbial group.

443. Pathogenicity: The condition or quality of being pathogenic, or the ability to cause disease.

444. Pathogenicity Island: A large segment of DNA in some pathogens that contains the genes responsible for virulence; often it codes for the type III secretion system that allows the pathogen to secrete virulence proteins and damage host cells. A pathogen may have more than one pathogenicity island.

445. Pathogenic Potential: The degree that a pathogen causes morbid signs and symptoms.

446. Ped: A natural soil aggregate, formed partly through bacterial and fungal growth in the soil.

447. Pencillins: A group of antibiotics containing a β-lactam ring, which are active against grampositive bacteria.

448. Peptic Ulcer Disease: A gastritis caused by Helicobacter pylori.

449. Peptidoglycan: A large polymer composed of long chain of alternating N-acetyl-glucosamine and N-acetylmuramic acid residues. The polysaccharide chains are linked to each other through connections between tetrapeptide chains attached to the N-acetylmuramic acids. It provides much of the strength and rigidity possessed by bacterial cell walls.

450. Peptones: Water-soluble digests or hydrolysates of proteins that are used in the preparation of culture media.

451. Period of Infectivity: Refers to the time during which the source of an infectious disease is infectious or is disseminating the pathogen.

452. Periplasmic Space or Periplasm: The space between the plasma membrane and the outer membrane in Gram-negative bacteria, and between the plasma membrane and the cell wall in Gram-positive bacteria.

453. Pertussis: An acute, highly contagious infection of the respiratory tract, most frequently affecting young children, usually caused by Bordetella pertussis or B. parapertussis. Consists of peculiar paroxysms of coughing, ending in a prolonged crowing or whooping respiration; hence the name whooping cough.

454. Petri Dish: A shallow dish consisting of two round, overlapping halves that is used to grow microorganisms on solid culture medium ; the top is larger than the bottom of the dish to prevent contamination of the culture.

455. Phase-contrast Microscope: A microscope that converts slight differences in refractive index and cell density into easily observed differences in light intensity.

456. Phenetic System: A classification system that groups organisms together based on the similarity of their observable characteristics.

457. Phenol Coefficient Test: A test to measure the effectiveness of disinfectants by comparing their activity against test bacteria with that of phenol.

458. Photolithotrophic Autorophs: Organisms that use light energy, an inorganic electron source (e.g., H_2O, H_2, H_2S) and CO_2 as a carbon source.

459. Photoorganotrophic Heterotrophs: Microorganisms that use light energy and organic electron donors, and also employ simple organic molecules rather than CO_2 as their carbon source.

460. Phototrophs: Organisms that use light as their energy source.

461. Phycobiliproteins: Photosynthetic pigments that are composed of proteins with attached tetrapyrroles; they are often found in cyanobacteria and red algae.

462. Phycobilisomes: Special particles on the membranes of cyanobacteria that contain photosynthetic pigments and electron transport chains.

463. Phylogenetic Tree: A graph made of nodes and branches, much like a tree in shape, that shows phylogenetic relationships between groups of organisms and sometimes also indicates the evolutionary development of groups.

464. Phytoplankton: A community of floating photosynthetic organisms, largely composed of algae and cyanobacteria.

465. Phytoremediation: The use of plants and their associated microorganisms to remove, contain, or degrade environmental contaminants.

466. Plankton: Free-floating, mostly microscopic microorganisms that can be found in almost all waters; a collective name.

467. Plaque: 1. A clear area in a lawn of bacteria or a localized area of cell destruction in a layer of animal cells that results from the lysis of the bacteria by bacteriophages or the destruction of the animal cells by animal viruses, 2. The term also refers to dental plaque, a film of food debris, polysaccharides, and dead cells that cover the teeth.

468. Plasmid Fingerprinting: A technique used to identify microbial isolates as belonging to the same strain because they contain the same number of plasmids with the identical molecular weights and similar phenotypes.

469. Plasmodial (acellular) Slime Mold: A member of the devision Myxomycota that exists as a thin, streaming, multinucleate mass of protoplasm which creeps along in an amoeboid fashion.

470. Plasmodium (pl. plasmodia): A stage in the life cycle of myxomycetes (plasmodial slime molds); a multinucleate mass of protoplasm surrounded by a membrane. Also, a parasite of the genus Plasmodium.

471. Plastid: A cytoplasmic orgenelle of algae and higher plants that contains pigments such as chlorophyll, stores food reserves, and often carries out processes such as photosynthesis.

472. Pleomorphic: Refers to bacteria that are variable in shape and lack a single, characteristic form.

473. Poly-β-hydroxybutyrate (PHB): A linear polymer of β-hydroxybutyrate used as a reserve of carbon and energy by many bacteria.

474. Polymerase Chain Reaction (PCR): An in vitro technique used to synthesize large quantities of specific nucleotide sequences from small amounts of DNA. It employs oligonucleotide primers complementary to specific sequences in the target gene and special heat-stable DNA polymerases.

475. Porin Proteins: Proteins that form channels across the outer membrane of Gram-negative bacterial cell walls. Small molecules are transported through these channels.

476. Pour Plate: A petri dish of solid culture medium with isolated microbial colonies growing both on its surface and within the medium, which has been prepared by mixing microorganisms with cooled, still liquid medium and then allowing the medium to harden.

477. Primary (frank) Pathogen: Any organism that causes a disease in the host by direct interaction with or infection of the host.

478. Primary Metabolites: Microbial metabolites produced during the growth phase of an organism.

479. Primary Producer: Photoautotrophic and chemoautotrophic organisms that incorporate carbon dioxide into organic carbon and thus provide new biomass for the ecosystem.

480. Primary Production: The incorporation of carbon dioxide into organic matter by photosynthetic organisms and chemoautotrophic bacteria.

481. Probiotic: A living organism that may provide health benefits beyond its nutritional value when it is ingested.

482. Procaryotic Cells: Cells that lack a true, membrane-enclosed nucleus; bacteria are procaryotic and have their genetic material located in a nucleoid.

483. Procaryotic Species: A collection of strains that share many stable properties and differ significantly from other groups of strains.

484. Propagated Epidemic: An epidemic that is characterized by a relatively slow and prolonged rise and then a gradual decline in the number of individuals infected. It usually results from the introduction of an infected individual into a susceptible population and the pathogen is transmitted from person to person.

485. Prostheca: An extension of a bacterial cell, including the plasma membrane and cell wall, that is narrower than the mature cell.

486. Protein Engineering: The rational design of proteins by constructing specific amino acid sequences through molecular techniques, with the objective of modifying protein characteristics.

487. Proteobacteria: A large group of bacteria, primarily Gram-negative, that 16S rRNA sequence comparisons show to be phylogenetically related; proteobacteria contain the purple photosynthetic bacteria and their relatives and are composed of the α, β, γ, δ and ε subgroups.

488. Proteome: The complete collection of proteins that an organism produces.

489. Protists: Eucaryotes with unicellular organization, either in the form of solitary cells or colonies of cells lacking true tissues.

490. Protoplast: A bacterial or fungal cell with its cell wall completely removed. It is spherical in shape and osmotically sensitive.

491. Protoplast Fusion: The joining of cells that have had their walls weakened or completely removed.

492. Prototroph: A microorganism that requires the same nutrients as the majority of naturally occurring members of its species.

493. Protozoan or Protozoon (Pl.Protozoa). A microorganism belonging to the Protozoa subkingdom. A unicellular or acellular eucaryotic protist whose organelles have the functional role of organs and tissues in more complex forms. Protozoa vary greatly in size, morphology, nutrition and life cycle.

494. Protozoology: The study of protozoa.

495. Pseudopodium or Pseudopod: A nonpermanent cytoplasmic extension of the cell body by which amoebae and amoeboid organisms move and feed.

496. Psittacosis (ornithosis): A disease due to a strain of Chlamydia psittaci, first seen in parrots and later found in other birds and domestic fowl (in which it is called ornithosis). It is transmissible to humans.

497. Psychrophile: A microorganisms that grows well at 0°C and has an optimum growth temperature of 15°C or lower and a temperature maximum around 20°C.

498. Psychrotroph: A microorganism that grows at 0°C, but has a growth optimum between 20 and 30°C and a maximum of about 35°C.

499. Puerperal Fever: An acute, febrile condition following childbirth; it is characterized by infection of the uterus and/or adjacent regions and is caused by streptococci.

500. Pulmonary Anthrax: A form of anthrax involving the lungs. Also known as woolsorter's disease.

501. Pure Culture: A population of cells that are identical because they arise from a single cell.

502. Putrefaction: The microbial decomposition of organic matter, especially the anaerobic breakdown of proteins, with the production of foul-smelling compounds such as hydrogen sulfide and amines.

503. Quellung Reaction: The increase in visibility or the swelling of the capsule of a microorganism in the presence of anitbodies against capsular antigens.

504. Quorum Sensing: The process in which bacteria monitor their own population density by sensing the levels of signal molecules that are released by the microorganisms. When these signal molecules reach a threshold concentration, quorum-dependent genes are expressed.

505. Rabies: An acute infectious disease of the central nervous system, which affects all warmblooded animals (including humans). It is caused by an ssRNA virus belonging to the genus Lyssavirus in the family Rhabdoviridae.

506. Radappertization: The use of gamma rays from a cobalt source for control of microorganisms in foods.

507. Radioimmunoassay (RIA): A very sensitive assay technique that uses a purified radioisotopelabeled antigen or antibody to compete for antibody or antigen with unlabeled standard and samples to determine the concentration of a substance in the samples.

508. Recombinant DNA Technology: The techniques used in carrying out genetic engineering; they involve the identification and isolation of a specific gene, the insertion of the gene into a vector such as a plasmid to form a recombinant molecule, and the production of large quantities of the gene and its products.

509. Recombinant-vector Vaccine: The type of vaccine that is produced by the introduction of one or more of a pathogen's genes into attenuated viruses or bacteria. The attenuated virus or bacterium serves as a vector, replicating within the vertebrate host and expressing the gene(s) of the pathogen. The pathogen's antigens induce an immune response.

510. Recombination: The process in which a new recombinant chromosome is formed by combining genetic material from two organisms.

511. Red Tides: Red tides occur frequently in coastal areas and often are associated with population blooms of dinoflagellates. Dinoflagellate pigments are responsible for the red colour of the water. Under these conditions, the dinoflagellates often produce saxitoxin, which can lead to paralytic shellfish poisoning.

512. Reductive Dehalogenation: The cleavage of carbon-halogen bonds by anaerobic bacteria that creates a strong electron-donating environment.

513. Regulatory Mutants: Mutant organisms that have lost the ability to limit synthesis of a product, which normally occurs by regulation of activity of an earlier step in the biosynthetic pathway.

514. Reservoir: A site, alternate host, or carrier that normally harbors pathogenic organisms and serves as a source from which other individuals can be infected.

515. Reservoir Host: An organism other than a human that is infected with a pathogen that can also infect humans.

516. Residuesphere: The region surrounding organic matter such as a seed or plant part in which microbial growth is stimulated by increased organic matter availability.

517. Resolution: The ability of a microscope to separate or distinguish between small objects that are close together.

518. Restricted Transduction: A transduction process in which only a specific set of bacterial genes are carried to another bacterium by a temperate phage; the bacterial genes are acquired because of a mistake in the excision of a prophage during the lysogenic life cycle.

519. Retroviruses: A group of viruses with RNA genomes that carry the enzyme reverse transcriptase and form a DNA copy of their genome during their reproductive cycle.

520. Ribotyping: Ribotyping is the use of E. coli rRNA to probe chromosomal DNA in Southern blots for typing bacterial strains. This method is based on the fact that rRNA genes are scattered throughout the chromosome of most bacteria and therefore polymorphic restriction endonuclease patterns result when chromosomes are digested and probed with rRNA.

521. Rocky Mountain Spotted Fever: A disease caused by Rickettsia rickettsii.

522. Root Nodule: Gall-like structures on roots that contain endosymbiotic nitrogen-fixing bacteria (e.g., Rhizobium or Bradyrhizobium is present in legume nodules).

523. Run: The straight line movement of a bacterium.

524. Salmonellosis: An infection with certain species of the genus Salmonella, usually caused by ingestion of food containing salmonellae or their products. Also known as Salmonella gastroenteritis or Salmonella food poisoning.

525. Sanitization: Reduction of the microbial population on an inanimate object to levels judged safe by public health standards; usually, the object is cleaned.

526. Saprophyte: An organism that takes up nonliving organic nutrients in dissolved form and usually grows on decomposing organic matter.

527. Saprozoic Nutrition: Having the type of nutrition in which organic nutrients are taken up in dissolved form; normally refers to animals or animal-like organisms.

528. Scanning Electron Microscope (SEM): An electron microscope that scans a beam of electrons over the surface of a specimen and forms an image of the surface from the electrons that are emitted by it.

529. Scanning Probe Microscope: A microscope used to study surface features by moving a sharp probe over the object's surface (e.g., the Scanning Tunneling Microscope).

530. Secondary Metabolites: Products of metabolism that are synthesized after growth has been completed.

531. Secondary Treatment: The biological degradation of dissolved organic matter in the process of sewage treatment ; the organic material is either mineralized or changed to settleable solids.

532. Selective Media: Culture media that favor the growth of specific microorganisms; this may be accomplished by inhibiting the growth of undesired microorganisms.

533. Selective Toxicity: The ability of a chemotherapeutic agent to kill or inhibit a microbial pathogen while damaging the host as little as possible.

534. Sepsis: Systemic response to infection. The systemic response is manifested by two or more of the following conditions as a result of infection : temperature > 38 or < 36 °C; heart rate > 90 beats per min; respiratory rate > 20 breaths per min, or pCO2 < 32 mm Hg; leukocyte count > 12,000 cells per ml3 or > 10% immature (band) forms. Sepsis also has been defined as the presence of pathogens or their toxins in blood and other tissues.

535. Septicemia: A disease associated with the presence in the blood of pathogens or bacterial toxins.

536. Septic Shock: Sepsis associated with severe hypotension despite adequate fluid resuscitation, along with the presence of perfusion abnormalities that may include, but are not limited to, lactic acidosis, oliguria, or an acute alternation in mental status. Gram-positive bacteria, fungi, and endotoxin-containing Gram-negative bacteria can initiate the pathogenic cascade of sepsis leading to septic shock.

537. Septum: A partition or crosswall that occurs between two cells in a bacterial (e.g. actinomycete or fungal filament, or which partitions off fungal structures such as spores. Septa also divide parent cells into two daughter cells during bacterial binary fission.

538. Serotyping: A technique or serological procedure that is used to differentiate between strains (serovars or serotypes) of microorganisms that have differences in the antigenic composition of a structure or product.

539. Serum (pl. Serums or Sera): The clear, fluid portion of blood lacking both blood cells and fibrinogen. It is the fluid remaining after coagulation of plasma, the noncellular liquid faction of blood.

540. Serum Resistance: The type of resistance that occurs with bacteria such as Neisseria gonorrhoeae because the pathogen interferes with membrane attack complex formation during the complement cascade.

541. Settling Basin: A basin used during water purification to chemically precipitate out fine particles, microorganisms, and organic material by coagulation or flocculation.

542. Sex Pilus: A thin protein appendage required for bacterial mating or conjugation. The cell with sex pili donates DNA to recipient cells.

543. Sheath: A hollow tubelike structure surroundings a chain of cells and present in several genera of bacteria.

544. Shigellosis: The diarrheal disease that arises from an infection with Shigella spp. Often called bacillary dysentery.

545. Shine-Dalgarno Sequence: A segment in the leader of procaryotic mRNA that binds to a special sequence on the 16S rRNA of the small ribosomal subunit. This helps properly orient the mRNA on the ribosome.

546. Shingles (Herpes Zoster): A reactivated form of chickenpox caused by the varicella-zoster virus.

547. Signal Peptide: The special amino-terminal sequence on a peptide destined for transport that delays protein folding and is recognized in bacteria by the Sec-dependent pathway machinery.

548. Silent Mutation: A mutation that does not result in a change in the organism's proteins or phenotype even though the DNA base sequence has been changed.

549. Simple Matching Coefficient (S SM): An association coefficient used in numerical taxonomy; the proportion of characters that match regardless of whether or not the attribute is present.

550. Site-specific Recombination: Recombination of nonhomologous genetic material with a chromosome at a specific site.

551. S-layer: A regularly structure layer composed of protein or glycoprotein that lies on the surface of many bacteria. It may protect the bacterium and help give it shape and rigidity.

552. Slime: The viscous extracellular glycoproteins or glycolipids produced by staphylococci and Pseudomonas aeruginosa bacteria that allows them to adhere to smooth surfaces such as prosthetic medical devices and catheters. More generally, ther term often refers to an easily removed, diffuse, unorganized layer of extracellular material that surrounds a bacterial cell.

553. Slime Layer: A layer of diffuse, unorganized, easily removed material lying outside the bacterial cell wall.

554. Slow Sand Filter: A bed of sand through which water slowly flows the gelatinous microbial layer on the sand grain surface removes waterborne microorganisms, particularly Giardia, by adhesion to the gel. This type of filter is used in some water purification plants.

555. Sorocarp: The fruiting structure of the Acrasiomycetes.

556. Sorus: A type of fruiting structure composed of a mass of spores or sporangia.

557. Source: The location or object from which a pathogen is immediately transmitted to the host, either directly or through an intermediate agent.

558. Species: Species of higher organisms are groups of interbreeding or potentially interbreeding natural populations that are reproductively isolated. Bacterial species are collections of strains that have many stable properties in common and differ significantly from other groups of strains.

559. Spheroplast: A relatively spherical cell formed by the weakening or partial removal of the rigid cell wall component (e.g., by pencillin treatment of Gram-negative bacteria). Spheroplasts are usually osmotically sensitive.

560. Spirillum: A rigid, spiral-shaped bacterium.

561. Spirochete: A flexible, spiral-shaped bacterium with periplasmic flagella.

562. Spore: A differentiated, specialized form that can be used for dissemiration, for survival of adverse conditions because of its heat and dessication resistance, and/or for reproduction. Spores are usually unicellular and may develop into vegetative organisms or gametes. They may be produced asexually or sexually and are of many types.

563. Sporulation: The process of spore formation.

564. Spread Plate: A petri dish of solid culture medium with isolated microbial colonies growing on its surface, which has been prepared by spreading a dilute microbial suspension evenly over the agar surface.

565. Stalk. A nonliving bacterial appendage produced by the cell and extending from it.

566. Staphylococcal Food Poisoning. A type of food poisoning caused by ingestion of improperly stored or cooked food in which Staphylococcus aureus has grown. The bacteria produce exotoxins that accumulate in the food.

567. Staphylococcal Scalded Skin Syndrome (SSSS): A disease caused by staphylococci that produce an exfoliative toxin. The skin becomes red (erythema) and sheets of epidermic may separate from the underlying tissue.

568. Starter Culture: An inoculum, consisting of a mixture of carefull selected microorganisms, used to start a commercial fermentation.

569. Stationary Phase: The phase of microbial growth in a batch culture when population growth ceases and the growth curve levels off.

570. Stem-nodulating Rhizobia: Rhizobia (members of the genera Rhizobium, Bradyrhizobium and Azorhizobium) that produce nitrogen-fixing structures above the soil surface on plant stems. These most often are observed in tropical plants and produced by Azorhizobium.

571. Sterilization: The process by which all living cells, viable spores, viruses, and viroids are either destroyed or removed from an objector habitat.

572. Strain: A population of organisms that descends from a single organism or pure culture isolate.

573. Streak Plate: A petri dish of solid culture medium with isolated microbial colonies growing on its surface, which has been prepared by spreading a microbial mixture over the agar surface, using an inoculating loop.

574. Streptococcal Pneumonia: A endogenous infection of the lungs caused by Streptococcus pneumoniae that occurs in predisposed individuals.

575. Streptococcal Sore Throat: One of the most common bacterial infections of humans. It is commonly referred to as "strep throat". The disease is spread by droplets of saliva or nasal secretions and is caused by Streptococcus spp. (particularly group A streptococci).

576. Streptolysin-O (SLO): A specific hemolysin produced by Streptococcus pyogenes that is inactivated by oxygen (hence the "O" in its name). SLO casuses beta-hemolysis of blood cells on agar plates incubated anaerobically.

577. Streptolysin-S (SLS): A product of Streptococcus pyogenes that is bound to the bacterial cell but may sometimes be released. SLS causes beta hemolysis on aerobically incubated blood-agar plates and can act as a leukocidin by killing leukocytes that phogocytose the bacterial cell to which it is bound.

578. Stromatolite: Dome-like microbial mat communities consisting of filamentous photosynthetic bacteria and occluded sediments (often calcareous or siliceous). They usually have a laminar structure. Many are fossilized, but some modern forms occur.

579. Superinfection: A new bacterial or fungal infection of a patient that is resistant to the drug(s) being used for treatment.

580. Swab: A wad of absorbent material usually wound around one end of a small stick and used for applying medication or for removing material from an area; also, a dacron-tipped polystyrene applicator.

581. Symbiosis: The living together or close association of two dissimilar organisms, each of these organisms being known as a symbiont.

582. Syntrophism: The association in which the growth of one organism either depends on, or is improved by, the provision of one or more growth factors or nutrients by a neighboring organism. Sometimes both organisms benefit.

583. Systematic Epidemiology: The field of epidemiology that focuses on the ecological and social factors that influence the development of emerging and reemerging infectious disease.

584. Systematics: The scientific study of organisms with the ultimate objective being to characterize and arrange them in an orderly manner ; often considered synonymous with taxonomy.

585. Taxon: A group into which related organisms are classified.

586. Taxonomy: The science of biological classification; it consists of three parts : classification, nomenclature and identification.

587. T Cell or T Lymphocyte: A type of lymphocyte derived from bone marrow stem cells that matures into an immunologically competent cell under the influence of the thymus. T cells are involved in a variety of cell-mediated immune reactions.

588. T-Cell Antigen Receptor (TCR): The receptor on the T cell surface consisting of two antigenbinding peptide chains ; it is associated with a large number of other glycoproteins. Binding of antigen to the TCR, usually in association with MHC, activates the T cell.

589. Teichoic Acids: Polymers of glycerol or ribitol joined by phosphates they are found in the cell walls of Gram-positive bacteria.

590. Temperate Phages: Bacteriophages that can infect bacteria and establish a lysogenic relationship rather than immediately lysing their hosts.

591. Tetanolysin: A hemolysin that aids in tissue destruction and is produced by Clostridium tetani.

592. Tetrapartite Associations: A symbiotic association of the same plant with three different types of microorganisms.

593. Theory: A set of principles and concepts that have survived rigorous testing and that provide a systematic account of some aspects of nature.

594. Thermal Death Time (TDT): The shortest period of time needed to kill all the organisms in a microbial population at a specified temperature and under defined conditions.

595. Thermoacidophiles: A group of bacteria that grow best at acid pHs and high temperatures; they are members of the Archaea.

596. Thermophile: A microorganism that can grow at temperatures of 55°C or higher; the minimum is usually around 45°C.

597. Thrush: Infection of the oral mucous membrane by the fungus Candila albicans; also known as oral candidiasis.

598. Toxigenicity: The capacity of an organism to produce a toxin.

599. Toxin: A microbial product or component that injures another cell or organism. Often the term refers to a poisonous protein, but toxins may be lipids and other substances.

600. Transformation: A mode of gene transfer in bacteria in which a piece of free DNA is taken up by a bacterial cell and integrated into the recipient genome.

601. Transgenic Animal or Plant: An animal or plant that has gained new genetic information from the insertion of foreign DNA. It may be produced by such techniques as injecting DNA into animal eggs, electroporation of mammalian cells and plant cell protoplasts, or shooting DNA into plants cells with a gene gun.

602. Transmission Electron Microscope (TEM): A microscope in which an image is formed by passing an electron beam through a specimen and focusing the scattered electrons with magnetic lenses.

603. Transovarian Passage: The passage of a microorganisms such as a rickettsia from generation to generation of hosts through tick eggs. (No humans or other mammals are needed as reservoirs for continued propagation.)

604. Traveller's Diarrhoea: A type of diarrhoea resulting from ingestion of viruses, bacteria, or protozoa normally absent from the traveller's environment. A major pathogen is enterotoxigenic Escherichia coli.

605. Trichomoniasis: A sexually transmitted disease caused by the parasitic protozoan Trichomonas vaginalis.

606. Tripartite Associations: A symbiotic association of the same plant with two types of microorganisms.

607. Trophozoite: The active, motile feeding stage of a protozoan organism; in the malarial parasite, the stage of schizogony between the ring stage and the schizont.

608. Tropism: The movement of living organisms toward or away from a focus of heat, light, or other stimulus.

609. Tubercle: A small, rounded nodular lesion produced by Mycobacterium tuberculosis.

610. Tuberculoid (neural) Leprosy: A mild, nonprogressive form of leprosy that is associated with delayed-type hypersensitivity to antigens on the surface of Mycobacterium leprae. It is characterized by early nerve damage and regions of the skin that have lost sensation and are surrounded by a border of nodules.

611. Tuberculosis (TB): An infectious disease of humans and other animals resulting from an infection by a species of Mycobacterium and characterized by the formation of tubercles and tissue necrosis, primarily as a result of host hypersensitivity and inflammation. Infection is usually by inhalation, and the disease commonly affects the lungs (pulmonary tuberculosis), although it may occur in any part of the body.

612. Tularemia: A plaguelike disease of animals caused by the bacterium Francisella tularensis subsp. tularensis (Jellison type A), which may be transmitted to humans.

613. Tumble: Random turning or tumbling movements made by bacteria when they stop moving in a striaght line.

614. Turbidostat: A continuous culture system equipped with a photocell that adjusts the flow of medium through the culture vessel so as to maintain a constant cell density or turbidity.

615. Ultramicrobacteria: Bacteria that can exist normally in a miniaturized form or which are capable of miniaturization under low-nutrient conditions. They may be 0.2 μm or smaller in diameter.

616. Ultraviolet (UV) Radiation: Radiation of fairly short wavelength, about 10 to 400 nm, and high energy.

617. Vector-borne Transmission: The transmission of an infectious pathogen between hosts by means of a vector.

618. Vehicle: An inanimate substance or medium that transmits a pathogen.

619. Vibrio: A rod-shaped bacterial cell that is curved to form a comma or an incomplete spiral.

620. Virology: The branch of microbiology that is concerned with viruses and viral diseases.

621. Virulence: The degree or intensity of pathogenicity of an organism as indicated by case fatality rates and/or ability to invade host tissues and cause disease.

622. Virulence Factor: A bacterial product, usually a protein or carbohydrate, that contributes to virulence or pathogenicity.

623. Virus: An infectious agent having a simple acellular oganization with a protein coat and a single type of nucleic acid, lacking independent metabolism and reproducing only within living host cells.

624. Vitamin: An organic compound required by organisms in minute quantities for growth and reproduction because it cannot be synthesized by the organism; vitamins often serve as enzyme cofactors or parts of cofactors.

625. Whole-genome Shotgun Sequencing: An approach to genome sequencing in which the complete genome is broken into random fragments, which are then individually sequenced. Finallly the fragments are placed in the proper order using sophisticated computer programs.

626. Whole-organism Vaccine: A vaccine made from complete pathogens, which can be of four types : inactivated viruses; attenuated viruses; killed microorganisms; and live, attenuated microbes.

627. Widal Test: A test involving agglutination of typhoid bacilli when they are mixed with serum containing typhoid antibodies from an individual having typhoid fever; used to detect the presence of Salmonella typhi and S. paratyphi.

628. Winogradsky Column: A glass column with an anaerobic lower zone and an aerobic upper zone, which allows growth of microorganisms under conditions similar to those found in a nutrient- rich lake.

629. Xenograft: A tissue graft between animals of different species.

630. Xerophilic Microorganisms: Microorganisms that grow best under low aw conditions and may not be able to grow at high aw values.

631. Yellow Fever: An acute infectious disease caused by a flavivirus, which is transmitted to humans by mosquitoes. The liver is affected and the skin turns yellow in this disease.

632. YM Shift: The change in shape by dimorphic fungi when they shift from the yeast (Y) form in the animal body to the mold or mycelial form (M) in the environment.

■ SUGGESTED READING

1. Introduction to Microbiology: A Case-History Study Approach (with CD-ROM and InfoTrac) by John L. Ingraham, Catherine A. Ingraham, Publisher: Brooks Cole, 2003.
2. Microbiology: An Introduction, Eighth Edition by Gerard J. Tortora, Berdell R. Funke, Christine L. Case, Publisher: Benjamin Cummings, 2003.
3. Microbiology: A Laboratory Manual (7th Edition) by James Cappuccino, Natalie Sherman, Publisher: Benjamin Cummings, 2013.
4. Sherris Medical Microbiology: An Introduction to Infectious Diseases by Kenneth J. Ryan, C. George Ray, Publisher: McGraw-Hill Medical, 2011.
5. Mims' Medical Microbiology by Richard Goering, Publisher: Elsevier, 2012.
6. Clinical Microbiology Made Ridiculously simple by M Gladwin, Publisher: Medmaster, 2014.
7. Cellular and Molecular Immunology by Abul K. Abbas, Publisher: Saunders, 2011.
8. Microbiology: Lippincott Illustrated Reviews Series by Richard A. Harvey Cynthia Nau Cornelissen, Publisher: Lippincott Williams & Wilkins, 2012.
9. Medical Microbiology by Patrick R. Murray, Publisher: Elsevier, 2012.
10. Medical Microbiology and Infection at a Glance by Stephen Gillespie, Publisher: Wiley-Blackwell, 2012.
11. Jawetz Melnick & Adelbergs Medical Microbiology by Geo. F. Brooks, Publisher: McGraw-Hill Medical, 2013.

Index

Page numbers followed by *f* refer to figure and *t* refer to table.